Bell's Palsy Handbook

Facial Nerve Palsy or Bell's Palsy Facial Paralysis Causes, Symptoms, Treatment, Face Exercises & Recovery All Covered

Alan McDonald

Disclaimer

This book contains information on Bell's palsy However; it is not intended to replace the advice of a licensed physician or healthcare professional. The book talks about Bell's palsy facial palsy and facial paralysis in general, not any specific person.

The author and publisher in any case will not be responsible for personal and commercial damages that result from the use of information, ideas, guidelines and suggestions mentioned herein. Please consult with a healthcare professional to address your specific concerns.

While utmost care has been taken to ensure the accuracy of the information published, it should only be used to inform yourself about the available choices. Treatment protocols featured within this publication are subject to change as new medical research and data emerges. If you wish to embark on any dietary, drug or lifestyle style, please seek clearance from your healthcare professional first.

The author will not be liable for damages of any kind arising from the use of this book. Also, the publisher and other people concerned with the development of this resource do not guarantee the authenticity and accuracy of information, ideas, and guidelines provided herein.

All content provided in or through the book is not intended or designed to promote or endorse any specific medical practice, treatment, diagnostic tests or procedures.

This book should not affect your consultation with practicing medical professionals. Do not rely solely on what you have read. Consult a certified healthcare professional for more information regarding your specific condition. **The author in no case recommends self-diagnosis and self-treatment.**

It is presumed that all readers have read the disclaimer and agree to all the facts mentioned facts before reading the book.

Acknowledgements

I would like to start off by thanking my parents. Without their support, I would not have been able to reach my goals and aspirations. They always enabled and inspired me to become a better human being and a better professional. Mom & Dad – you are my true inspiration. Thank you for helping me get through the most difficult phase of my life. I will cherish your guidance and encouragement forever.

I would also like to thank Dr. Alexa Smith, MD for her valuable contributions that have helped me write this comprehensive and holistic book on Bell's palsy. Dr. Smith, your advice on both research and the contents of this book are invaluable.

Special thanks go out to all my friends for supporting me and encouraging me throughout this writing experience.

Preface

I have always been a firm believer that every human being is put on this Earth to fulfill his or her destiny and contribute to society in his or her own way. While there will always be certain obstacles that momentarily prevent us from achieving greatness, with dedication and commitment, we can always emerge victorious in the end.

My life has been no different, filled with battles at various stages in life – one of the biggest battles being Bell's palsy. At 34, I'm having the time of my life. But having to deal with "Bell's Palsy" wasn't always easy. I knew I had to be strong to fit in and define my presence in this world. I wish that this book existed when I first started looking for information on Bell's palsy. I had to scour through countless books, message boards and various other literature to find valuable information on this condition back then. That's why I have written this book, which contains everything you need to know about Bell's palsy, all in one place.

Earlier in my life, I couldn't be bothered about how my face looked or what anyone said about me. Like every other happy-go-lucky child, I was busy having fun and looking forward to my next trip to the park.

Unfortunately, Bell's palsy is a condition that you firstly can't hide and secondly, cannot be oblivious about. A drooping face is certainly not normal for anyone to have or see. Staying in foster care didn't help much and there was barely any improvement in my condition. I'm grateful to my parents who adopted me at 11 months and brought me home. Today, after 34 years, I don't want to blame anyone. What would have happened had I received timely medical attention? Would this condition have gone away in a few weeks? Was there a chance of full recovery? I really don't know the answers.

But what I do know is that I'm writing this book to let people know that vast improvement, even 100% recovery is possible with the right treatment and management procedures. With great advancement in medicine and various treatment options available, you may not have to live with Bell's palsy forever.

Most of the time, I don't even think of my palsy as a disadvantage because it taught me to exhibit other strengths of mine. However, my journey wasn't the smoothest. My insecurities were real. The issue was that I had a huge adjustment to make. What I saw in the mirror was a person with an unusual smile. I was worried when I stepped outside to meet new people. I felt uncomfortable, and, therefore, avoided getting photographs taken since I had trouble controlling my facial expressions.

It might seem bizarre to you, but not all people want to befriend a person with a collapsed face. The impact Bell's palsy has on a person's self-confidence, and self-esteem is undoubtedly devastating. With this condition, you always stand out from the crowd, and many people don't fully understand it, which is why they may try to avoid it or you altogether.

Because I grew up with the condition, I want others with the same ailment to know that there is light at the end of the tunnel. There is no need to feel isolated because I'll teach you how to cope with Bell's palsy, from understanding the condition, to managing and treating it, and knowing how to act and react around others.

Don't be saddened by any negative comments thrown your way. Remember, you can still stand strong without the validation of others. It is comforting to know that people who suffer from Bell's palsy can completely recover from the condition. This means they can fully control their facial expressions again. However, there's a lot to learn about this ailment before making an effort to cure it or deal with it. So let's get going and develop a clearer picture about the causes, symptoms, treatment and management of Bell's palsy.

Contents

Chapter One: Introduction

What Do We Know about Bell's Palsy?

The Science behind the Name

The term Bell's palsy comes from Sir Charles Bell, a renowned 19th century Scottish anatomist and surgeon who discovered that the condition is caused by the dysfunction of the 7th facial nerve.

The Facial Nerve

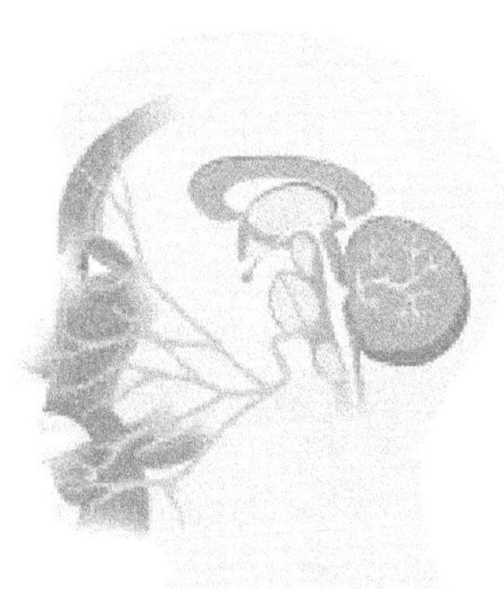

Sir Charles Bell

Born in Scotland in 1774, Sir Charles Bell studied anatomy and medicine at the legendary University of Edinburgh. He and his brother left for London after being rejected by the Edinburgh Royal Infirmary.

Sir Charles Bell returned to Scotland after living and working in London for almost 30 years. He ended his teaching career as a professor of surgery at the place he studied – University of Edinburgh. Bell also was an expert surgeon. In fact in 1815, he served in the British Army at the famous Battle of Waterloo. He's also recognized for his medical illustration in neurology. The essays written by Sir Charles Bell on the anatomy of expression in painting are still considered a classic piece of art history.

Is There a Difference between Facial Paralysis and Bell's Palsy?

People who lose the ability to move one side of their face are said to be victims of 'facial paralysis.' It is a general term and is frequently used when the facial muscles become paralyzed due to the facial nerve being injured. Facial paralysis also occurs when the facial nerve suffers any kind of trauma through a stroke, infection, or tumor.

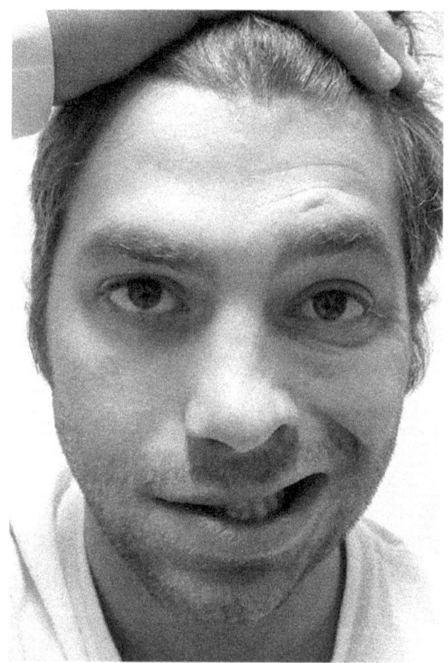

Credit: *'Bell's palsy' by James Heilman MD from Wikipedia Commons (https://commons.wikimedia.org/wiki/File:Bellspalsy.JPG) under the Creative Commons Attribution-Share Alike 3.0 Unported License*

Facial paralysis is characterized by a non-symmetrical face; the person is unable to move some/all of the muscles on the affected side. Since facial muscles cannot be controlled in paralysis, routine activities such as chewing, sipping, swallowing and speaking become difficult.

Bell's palsy perhaps, is the most common form of facial paralysis you will come across. We will discuss the symptoms, causes, and diagnosis of Bell's palsy in detail later in the book, but for now remember this.

Bell's palsy patients have facial paralysis, but not everyone with facial paralysis has Bell's palsy. A person is diagnosed with Bell's palsy only when facial paralysis is not associated with any medical condition such as stroke, autoimmune disease, trauma or tumor.

What Really Happens?

The term 'palsy' in Bell's palsy generally refers to the weakness of facial muscles. When your facial nerve stops functioning, the muscles in your face fail to receive the much-needed electrical signals to function properly. This lack of 'electrical communication' results in paralysis of the affected side of the face – this may include your eyes, mouth as well as other facial muscles. What's scary about it is the fact that this loss of facial muscle control (facial paralysis) occurs rapidly - it can even happen overnight!

Sadly, medical research cannot predict the degree or extent of facial paralysis or muscle weakness. Quite often, only the lower half of the face is affected. At times, Bell's palsy can affect the whole side of the face or even worse, both sides of the face can become paralyzed. Bell's palsy on both sides of the face, however, is extremely rare. Now moving forward, let's see what the muscles in our face can do.

The Muscles Used for Facial Expressions

You will be surprised with the long list of functions your facial muscles perform. The 7th cranial nerve is responsible for controlling the following muscles and their corresponding functions.

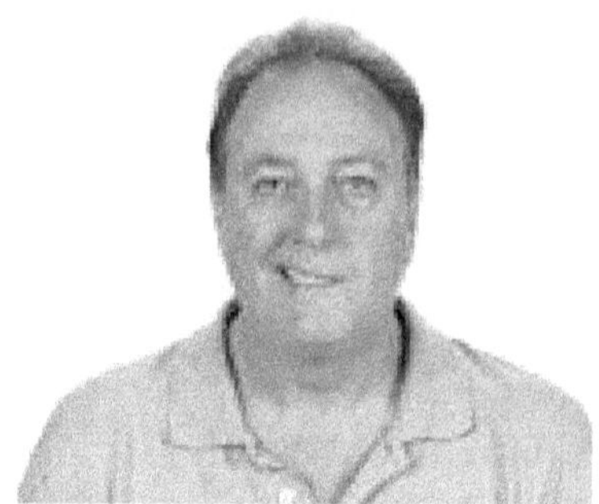

1) Occipitofrontalis muscle – raising the eyebrows

2) Zygomaticus – raises the corners of the mouth during 'open mouth' smiling. Surprisingly, a variation in the structure of this muscle causes 'dimples.'

3) Risorius – Closed mouth smiling

4) Corrugator supercilii – frowning

5) Orbicularis oculi – closing the eyes

6) Orbicularis oris – used for closing the mouth and 'pouting'

7) Levator labii – lifting upper lip

8) Depressor labii – helps pull lower lip down

9) Mentalis – helps stick bottom lip out

10) Nasalis – helps 'wrinkle' the nose

Can I Predict My Chances?

Bell's palsy affects 0.02% of the population. The incidence increases with age and people with certain medical conditions are simply more prone than others. The disorder has been linked to cold sores, flu-like illness, diabetes, tumors, skull and facial injuries and Lyme disease.

Bell's palsy, as we've discussed, tends to appear suddenly out of the blue – symptoms may start appearing without even the slightest warning. So you may go to bed with a perfectly symmetrical face and when you wake up the next morning; you may notice that your face has collapsed on one side.

Some people feel numbness or weakness in their facial muscles a day or two before the symptoms first appear. If you notice pain behind your ear or normal sounds seem uncomfortably loud, do get it checked immediately.

The signs and symptoms of Bell's palsy tend to reach their peak within a day or two after appearing. Most patients feel that they are having a stroke, but here's something you need to remember. In the case of stroke, muscle weakness is also felt in other parts of the body, not just your face.

Prognosis and Chances of Recovery

The prognosis for Bell's palsy is generally good; however, recovery times may vary from person to person. The extent of nerve damage is what determines how soon the condition will go away. Most people start to get better within two weeks with complete recovery in about 3 to 6 months. A small number of people may take longer to recover.

The National Health Service UK states that 7 out of 10 people make a complete recovery. As mentioned earlier, the time will depend on the amount of nerve damage. The remaining 3 out of 10 people are stuck with the condition in severe cases, however, the majority of cases are treatable.

What about Recurrence?

In rare cases, Bell's palsy may recur either on the same or the opposite side of the face and why it does so is another guessing game. Again, potential viruses might have an important role to play.

The following is a list of infections that might cause a recurrence of Bell's palsy.

1) Cold sores
2) Genital herpes
3) Chickenpox
4) Shingles
5) Epstein-Barr syndrome
6) Cytomegalovirus infections
7) Respiratory illnesses, particularly upper respiratory tract infections
8) Rubella
9) Mumps
10) Influenza

The bad news is that the herpes simplex virus, adenovirus, and herpes zoster virus cannot be eradicated from the body even after you are cured. Simply put, if you had chicken pox, measles or mumps at a young age, the virus may remain dormant for years and reactivate suddenly to cause Bell's palsy. This, however, doesn't mean you will necessarily be affected.

Living with the Condition:

Bell's palsy is rarely counted as a life-threatening condition, but it is certainly socially difficult to endure. The characteristic one-sided facial droop slowly worms its way into the subconscious of the sufferer and creates persistent feelings of hopelessness and being 'socially unacceptable.' These insidious feelings affect all kinds of interactions from personal relationships to your circle of friends and even boardroom presentations.

What makes Bell's palsy so baffling is that researchers are still trying to determine the exact cause. Moreover, there is no vaccine for prevention. However, all is not lost since we already know that the condition can be treated.

I can understand the feelings of abandonment, but remember; there is hope. I never received the recommended treatment in foster care. Additionally, being bullied at school took a toll on my social life. It was a frightening time for me because I felt like an outcast with only a few friends. I had a hard time overcoming the thought that most people didn't want to spend time with me.

Despite the fact that most people with Bell's palsy are highly social and love to make new friends, they may prefer 'staying behind closed doors'. I too felt the same way at a young age, but things are different now. The love and support of my parents helped me overcome hurdles and lead a good life. Today, facial paralysis does not stop me from being 'myself.'

Who Can Be Affected?

Bell's palsy is listed as a rare medical occurrence that only occurs in 1 in 5,000 people every year. It can strike anyone; either men or women aged between 15 and 45 years are more commonly affected.

In the past, Bell's palsy was simply thought to be a case of unusual appearance. Since viral infections may cause the condition, it is more likely to affect individuals with a compromised immune system.

Bell's palsy sadly is also rated as the most common cause of one-sided facial muscle weakness in children. However, the majority of sufferers are adults.

The severity of symptoms or recovery rate doesn't seem to vary a great deal across both genders. Neither does race nor ethnicity make a difference as far as being at risk is concerned. So the good news is that regardless of where your ancestors are from, you are not specifically more at risk to get Bell's palsy. However, the flip side is that since the disease has no bounds, anyone can be affected by it.

Are You at Risk?

About 40,000 people are affected with the disorder in the United States annually. While Bell's palsy can happen at almost any age, studies have identified groups that are at higher risk for developing the condition.

1) Expecting Mothers

Pregnant women, especially during the third trimester of pregnancy or moms who have recently given birth are at greater risk of developing Bell's palsy. The condition however does not appear to have any effect on the developing fetus.

2) Diabetics

Diabetes is seen as a potential trigger for Bell's palsy. Researchers believe that the condition is related to the damage of blood vessels caused by diabetes.

3) Patients with upper respiratory tract infections

Patients with URIs, Upper Respiratory Tract Infections such as cold or flu are also at greater risk of developing Bell's palsy. The exact reason is unknown, but researchers have linked it to a weakened immune system that allows dormant viruses to attack the 7th cranial nerve.

Facing the Camera

List of celebrities with Facial palsy

George Clooney

Twice voted the 'Sexiest Man alive', Oscar winning actor George Clooney suffered from Bell's palsy while he was a freshman in high school. Fortunately, he recovered from the condition within a year. However, while recalling his time with the condition; the actor described it as the worst time of his life.

His schoolmates laughed at and mocked him. It was devastating as his left eye closed and he also faced difficulty eating and drinking properly. He got the nickname 'Frankenstein' during this period because of his face. But his experience with this condition made him stronger.

Pierce Brosnan

Famous for his dapper good looks and his role in the 'James Bond' film franchise, the Irish actor Pierce Brosnan had to battle Bell's palsy as well. He fell victim to the condition in 1984.

Facial paralysis occurred in the dressing room just before his appearance on an American show, namely the 'Tonight Show'. He failed to close one of his eyes and felt his face go numb, but the actor recovered from the condition within a few months.

Sylvester Stallone:

One of the greatest action stars of all times and best known for portraying Rocky, Sylvester Stallone is also a sufferer of Bell's palsy since birth. The condition was caused due to birth complications resulting in facial disfigurement and slurred speech. However, Stallone is an inspiration as he not only overcame his adversity, but also achieved greatness.

The use of forceps at birth had injured his nerve, paralyzing the lower left half of his face. However, this action hero used this to his advantage and today he is distinguished for his snarling look that has become his trademark.

Roseanne Barr

This Emmy award winning actress and acclaimed comedian was affected by Bell's palsy at the tender age of three. She describes in her autobiography that she felt as if her face had frozen. Barr's left side of her face was affected with the condition. Barr's case was that of temporary Bell's palsy, and she made a remarkably quick recovery.

Jim Ross

Known as the voice of WWE, the famous professional wrestling commentator has been fighting Bell's palsy since 1994. It was in 1998 that Ross's mother passed away, and the tragedy was followed by a second Bell's palsy attack.

In 2009, the WWE Hall of Famer was affected by a bout of Bell's palsy for the third time. His eyesight and right side of his face have been affected due to these attacks. The likes of Jim Ross are a source of encouragement for anyone battling Bell's palsy. He successfully conquered these health issues and achieved success and greatness.

Glenda McKay

This popular British actress is well known for her role in the popular UK television soap opera, Emmerdale, as 'Rachel Hughes'. In addition to being a talented actor, Glenda McKay is also a theater artist, teacher and a qualified aerobics instructor.

The Emmerdale star played her character from 1988 to 1999, and it was during the filming of this soap that she was diagnosed with Bell's palsy.

According to McKay, the onset of the condition was sudden. Whilst she was busy filming, the actress felt that her mouth had drooped. She thought it was a stroke possibly – sadly most patients mistaken a collapsed face for a stroke. Towards the end of the shoot, McKay recalls that the symptoms became worse. She was unable to apply lipstick and other makeup.

In various interviews, the actress commented that she was worried about her career ending abruptly and thought that the condition would remain with her for the rest of her life.

Fortunately for McKay, she began to recover within a few months. Steroid medication worked well for her and helped her condition improve tremendously.

Rick Savage

Brilliant bassist and member of the renowned metal band Def Leppard, Rick Savage is another celebrity who dealt with Bell's palsy. Popularly known as 'Sav,' Rick was extremely popular among female fans largely because of his good looks. He was also called the pretty boy of this English band.

In 1994, Rick Savage was diagnosed with Bell's palsy. The condition 'froze' one side of his face and his facial muscles weakened. According to Savage, his face felt as if it had melted. His reputation as a sex symbol received a serious blow. He resorted to various treatments including steroids, but he believes it was acupuncture that helped him recover rapidly.

Rick Savage has managed to recover from this condition, but some symptoms are still visible. These effects can be observed clearly when he seems fatigued and weary. Rick once commented that it was difficult to not be able to do everyday things such as eat properly and not sleep without covering his eye with an eye patch. However, Rick also had to witness the tragedy that his fellow band member Rick Allen went through when he lost his arm. This helped Savage deal with his condition.

Alexis Denisof

Alexis Denisof is a famous American actor who has worked extensively in theater, television productions as well as movies. However, he is largely recognized for his great role in 'Buffy the Vampire Slayer', a television series.

In 1999, three weeks before the filming of 'Angel' Season Five, Alexis was affected by Bell's palsy. According to Joss Whedon, who was directing the series, Denisof found it hard to speak and move the left side of his face, which was paralyzed due to the condition.

The actor was concerned that he would not be able to shoot the first episode properly. However, he began to recover by that time, but considering the immobility problem with his left side, the director chose to do things differently. Most of Denisof's shots were kept on his right side during the filming of the episode.

Ralph Nader

Included in Time Magazine's list of 100 Most Influential Americans in the Twentieth Century, Ralph Nader is not just a political activist. He is one of the top consumer advocates, an author and a lawyer.

The reason he is included in our list is that Nader has also suffered from Bell's palsy. The 1980s were difficult for him. In 1986, he lost his older brother who died of prostate cancer. In the same phase, Ralph Nader developed this condition which adversely affected the left side of his face.

For several months, Nader had to put up with half of his face being paralyzed and a droopy eyelid. Due to Bell's palsy, he also suffered from excessive tearing and could not blink his left eye. Nader started wearing sunglasses to hide these effects, but he dealt with the condition fearlessly.

Graeme Garden

Famous British television presenter, comedian, actor and author, Graeme Garden was also diagnosed with Bell's palsy. In December

2002, Garden felt some changes in his face. He commented that he was unable to whistle. And after that he noticed that the left side of his face started to go numb.

Garden, while recalling his experience with this condition commented that it became embarrassing to eat and drink. Smiling too became uncomfortable for him because it looked like a half smile rather than a full one.

He also pointed out that it was tremendously difficult to articulate sounds, especially the sounds of the letter F and P. However; he managed to recover from the condition down the road.

Jean Chretien

Jean Chretien served as the Prime Minister of Canada from 1993-2003. Apart from his political career, he is also a renowned lawyer and author. The former Canadian Prime Minister developed Bell's palsy at a very young age, when he was merely 12 years old. Unfortunately, that resulted in permanent paralysis of the left side of his face.

Although Bell's palsy improves within weeks or months in most people, certain individuals might suffer from lingering effects and Chretien's case is one example. It was never easy for a boy entering his teen years to experience a droopy and numb face. However, even after being afflicted by Bell's palsy, Jean Chretien excelled in life and went on to become Canada's 20th Prime Minister. He is also the recipient of several prestigious awards and honors.

Chapter Two: Causes, Symptoms and Diagnosis

This particular section gives a more detailed description of the anatomy of the 7th cranial nerve to help you understand the disorder.

Anatomy of the 7th Cranial Nerve

Facial muscles control the expressions of your face, from making you smile to making you frown. This is why these muscles are so important, since they help us understand each other better and decipher non-verbal cues. These muscles are controlled by the facial nerve, also known as the 7th cranial nerve.

The 7th nerve branches out from the brainstem into an extremely narrow canal in your skull called the Fallopian canal. It then exits the skull at a point right behind your ear. The anatomy, as you can guess is not so simple. The 7th nerve then spreads out from behind the ear and splits into several branches to control the muscles on each side of the face.

What are the Known Causes?

Some viruses are thought to cause Bell's palsy but what exactly triggers the response is unknown. Studies suggest that environmental factors, trauma, stress and metabolic disorders might contribute to the reactivation of the already existing 'dormant virus.' The nerve swells and becomes inflamed in response to the viral infection – this is one of the reasons steroids are known to reduce inflammation and swelling, and are useful in treating Bell's palsy.

Other popular treatment methods include:

a. Antiviral medications to treat viral infection

b. Analgesics or painkillers to relieve pain (if present)

c. Physical therapy to stimulate the affected facial nerve

Alternative treatments used include:

a. Electrical stimulation

b. Acupuncture

c. Vitamin B therapy

d. Biofeedback therapy

e. Facial rehabilitation

Your physiotherapist will also teach you a number of facial exercises that will strengthen the muscles in your face. Physical exercises have shown impressive results in improving coordination and the range of 'facial muscle' movement.

Why does a dormant virus attack that nerve in particular? This is something scientists are working day and night to try and figure out.

How Do Your Facial Nerves Work?

Each side of your face is controlled by its own facial nerve. Simply put, if your left 7th cranial nerve is affected, the effects will be seen only on the left side of your face.

The 7th cranial nerve allows you to move your forehead, close your eyelids, blink your eye, open and close your mouth and smile and frown.

Other important functions of the 7th cranial nerve include carrying impulses to a small muscle in your middle ear and controlling saliva and tear production. The amount of saliva you secrete and the volume at which you perceive sound is also controlled directly by the 7th cranial nerve.

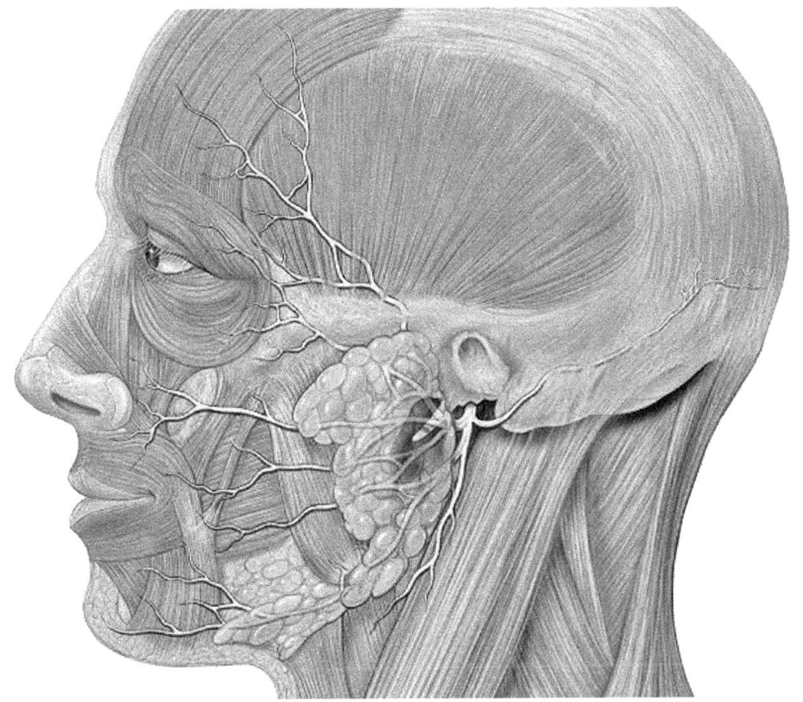

Credit: *'Facial Nerve' by Maen K. Housen from Wikipedia Commons (https://commons.wikimedia.org/wiki/File:Head_facial_nerve_branches.jpg) under the Creative Commons Attribution-Share Alike 3.0 Unported License*

Research shows that the facial nerve is also responsible for taste sensations in the tongue. Interestingly, taste sensations in two-thirds of your tongue are also sent to the brain via the same nerve.

It is estimated that the 7th cranial nerve branches into 7000 nerve fibers to control a wide range of facial muscle and neck activity. As mentioned earlier, a healthy facial nerve is responsible for maintaining healthy facial muscles.

Symptoms of Bell's Palsy

Since a critical controlling nerve is out of order in Bell's palsy, the forehead smoothens and the corner of the mouth droops. The eyelid does not close on the affected side, and eye irritation often results from continuous exposure to air and external elements. Patients also complain of food and saliva spilling from the affected corner of the mouth.

The characteristic drooping of the mouth is upsetting since it makes your face look 'different'. Along with facial paralysis, Bell's palsy patients may experience a loss of taste on the affected side. Some patients also report hearing sounds louder than usual, and this is often accompanied with pain in the ear area.

How Does Bell's Palsy Affect Facial Muscle Function?

The symptoms can vary greatly among different patients, but here is a quick overview of what may happen.

Forehead

You may lose the ability to wrinkle your forehead and frown

Effects on the Eyes include:

1) Sensitivity to light
2) Inability to raise eyebrow/eyebrows
3) Droopy eyebrows
4) Drooping of lower eyelid
5) Inability to close eyelid fully
6) Inability to blink
7) Inability to squint
8) Tearing
9) Dry eyes

10) Redness and soreness in the sclera – the white part of the eye

11) Irritation and pain in the eyes

12) Please note: seek medical help immediately if you are experiencing any problems with your eyes.

Mouth

1) Corner of the mouth droops or pulls down
2) Difficulty speaking
3) Difficulty smiling, eating and drinking
4) Inability to whistle or blow out air
5) Altered taste sensation, can be accompanied with tingling sensations on the affected side of the tongue
6) Difficulty opening mouth, brushing, flossing and spitting
7) Dry mouth
8) Changes in quantities of saliva produced
9) Inability to pull the lips back or pout

Ears

1) Sensitivity to sound
2) Pain in the affected ear or behind the ear
3) Loss of hearing

Nose

1) Inability to flare nostrils

2) Inability to wrinkle nose

What Causes Bell's Palsy?

While it does sound shocking, doctors still don't know the exact cause of the ailment. What's even more surprising is that people are diagnosed with the condition after the doctor is unable to figure out what caused facial paralysis in the first place.

Medical expert's suspect that viral infections such as those caused by the herpes virus lead to the swelling of the 7th cranial nerve. This inflammation and swelling of the 7th nerve disrupts the signals sent from and to facial muscles.

Other factors such as herpes zoster virus (responsible for chickenpox), mononucleosis (Epstein-Barr syndrome), emotional stress and environmental factors can cause inflammation of the facial nerve, therefore, they are also listed as potential causes.

Stress and lack of sleep have been linked to the reactivation of the herpes virus. Prolonged stress or emotional trauma can also weaken the immune system, which gives the herpes virus a chance to grow stronger and infect the nerve.

There are different types of herpes viruses that can cause irritation and swelling of the facial nerve. These include the herpes simplex virus (HSV), including herpes type 1, which causes cold sores, herpes type 2 which causes genital herpes and varicella-zoster virus, which causes chickenpox and shingles.

The Herpes family or Herpes viruses share some common characteristics. They have a long life, and perhaps the most dangerous trait is going into a dormant phase. Shockingly, the herpes viruses can remain dormant for decades after the initial infection. The reason 60-70% of Bell's palsy cases show signs of herpes infection is that the viruses have a special affinity for nerve tissue.

Simply put, you might not be aware that the herpes virus is present inside your body.

HSV-1 in particular is a virus several people have been exposed to. It can easily spread through kissing or sharing utensils and towels. Medical researchers are amazed by the diversity of infections herpes viruses cause. You will be surprised to know that chickenpox, cold sores and sexually transmitted diseases are all caused by Herpes viruses.

Diagnosis

While Bell's palsy is believed to be caused by the inflammation of the facial nerve, other conditions can produce facial paralysis identical to what you observe in a sudden Bell's palsy attack.

You should visit the nearest hospital or call an ambulance immediately if you or someone around you develops facial paralysis. Studies have shown that Bell's palsy can be managed more effectively if the treatment is started within 72 hours of the development of the first symptoms.

The doctor will ask you in detail about your medical history and perform a thorough examination to determine the cause. Usually, the questions and diagnostic tests help doctors rule out the possibility of other conditions that can cause facial paralysis.

Conditions that Need to Be Ruled Out

Several other conditions, as mentioned earlier, also result in facial paralysis. This is the most striking characteristic of Bell's palsy. Your doctor will recommend a series of tests and look for any evidence that might confirm that your symptoms point towards Bell's palsy.

Here are some medical conditions that might cause facial nerve paralysis:

1. Lyme disease: a particular bacterial infection caused by ticks. Patients with Lyme disease also complain about rashes and joint pain.

   This disease is common in North America and Europe. Deer ticks, which feed on the blood of animals and humans, play an important part in spreading the bacteria 'Borrelia burgdorferi'. The risk of getting infected is more if you spend a great deal of time in grassy or woody areas. You also need to be extra careful if you live in an area where Lyme disease is prevalent.

2. Moebius syndrome: a rare congenital birth defect.
3. Abnormal tissue growth or tumors.
4. Stroke.
5. Middle ear infections.
6. Cholesteatoma – unusual collection of skin cells in the middle ear.
7. Head and skull injuries.

Physical Evaluation

Your doctor will examine your head, ears and neck closely. This physical examination will also include careful inspection of the ear canal, salivary glands and facial muscles. Your doctor will check the muscles in your face to confirm whether only the facial nerve has been affected with palsy. If there is no evidence of other medical conditions, your doctor will confirm Bell's palsy. However, further diagnostic tests may be recommended before starting treatment.

Frequently Asked Questions

Your doctor may ask a series of questions for further evaluation of your condition. Below are the most likely questions you can expect during your visit.

1. Are your facial muscles feeling weak?
2. Can you close your eyelids completely?
3. Do you have watery eyes?

4. Can you raise your eyebrows?

5. Do you have ear pain? If so, on which side?

6. Do you have problems hearing?

7. Have you had problems chewing?

8. Is there any change in your sense of taste?

9. When did your symptoms develop?

10. Have you had an upper respiratory tract infection, for example, a cold recently?

11. Have you been vaccinated recently?

Questions You Can Ask Your Doctor

1. Are there any other symptoms I should look out for?

2. What tests will be involved in diagnosing my condition?

3. What will these tests tell me?

4. Are diagnostic tests painful?

5. How long will the tests take?

6. When will I know the test's results?

7. Will I need more tests?

8. What are my treatment options?

9. Do I need to come for a follow-up visit and if so, when?

10. Do I need to take any precautions?

Further Diagnostic Testing

In case your doctor is still uncertain, you may be referred to an ear, nose and throat (ENT) specialist and a neurologist for further testing. You may have to get electromyography and imaging scans to check for facial nerve damage and complications.

Your doctor may also suggest the following lab tests:

a. Hearing test if you have problems hearing

b. Computed tomography scan of the head if your medical history and condition show signs of a stroke or tumor

Electromyography

During electromyography (EMG), a very thin needle will be inserted to pass a mild electric current through the skin and into your facial muscle. A machine called an oscilloscope then measures the electrical activity in your muscles and nerves. Though the test doesn't sound pleasant, it is not very painful. This information is useful to assess the extent of any nerve damage if present.

EMG measures the difference between the two action potentials generated by your facial muscles on both sides of the face. These potentials are generated in response to the stimulation of the facial nerve by the tiny electric current.

Imaging Scans

Imaging scans including MRIs and a CT scan of the brain may be recommended to make sure that your problem (facial paralysis) is not caused by a stroke, an infection or a tumor. The doctor usually detects other signs of stroke, infections and tumors during the physical examination. A facial CT scan may be used to rule out possibilities of facial fractures.

Chapter Three: Kid's Health and Facial Palsy

Although Bell's palsy is more common in adults, children and adolescents can also fall victim to it.

The condition affects children in a different manner because they are often unable to understand why it has come about or how to treat it. However, children too can recover completely and quickly when given timely treatment. Sadly, a very small number of young children may suffer from the disease permanently.

Bell's Palsy Causes in Children

People may assume that most Bell's palsy causes are the same in children as they are in adults. However, this is not always true. Bell's palsy in children isn't common, but it occurs due to a variety of factors. It is believed that when the facial nerve becomes inflamed or swollen, the irritation causes Bell's palsy. However, the specific trigger for inflammation is not established. The different reasons that may cause this condition in children and teenagers are:

1) Birth trauma:

Infants can fall victim to Bell's palsy as a result of trauma during birth. This could happen due to a difficult forceps delivery in several cases.

2) Viral Infection:

Research links Bell's palsy with viral infections such as herpes, which is known to cause cold sores. The herpes virus however is just one suggested trigger. Several other viruses are believed to play an important part in triggering the inflammatory response.

3) Infectious diseases:

Lyme disease is also one of the causes of Bell's palsy in children, especially those living in wooded areas. It is worth noting that not everyone who gets affected by these infectious diseases or infections develops Bell's palsy. A lot of kids don't. Therefore, washing hands should be a regular practice among children so that the spread of viruses can be prevented.

4) Injury to the face:

An injury or head trauma (such as skull fracture) causing damage to the facial nerve can also cause this condition in children.

5) Middle Ear Infection, Diabetes:

Children who have diabetes are prone to flu and cold, and those with a compromised immune system are at a greater risk of being affected by Bell's palsy.

6) Tumor:

A tumor could exert pressure on the facial nerve, thereby triggering Bell's palsy in kids. In the case of a blood clot, a stroke could also cause Bell's palsy to develop in children.

Symptoms of Bell's Palsy in Children

The signs and symptoms of this condition differ from person to person and vary in severity from mild weakness to paralysis in one or both sides of the face.

Symptoms of Bell's palsy show up suddenly. Sometimes, they begin gradually and could take a period of a few days or even weeks. However, it is seen that most symptoms that appear unexpectedly tend to peak in almost 48 hours.

If your kid is showing any of these symptoms, contact your health practitioner without any delay.

a. Pain around the jaw

b. Stiffness or twitching on the affected side of the face

c. Trouble closing the eye on the affected side

d. Difficulty smiling

e. Drooping of the corner of the mouth or eyelid

f. Trouble eating and drinking

g. Changes in the amount of tears and saliva

h. Headache

i. Trouble speaking, causing slurred speech

j. Earache. There is also hypersensitivity to sound in the affected ear

k. Numbness of the mouth

l. Strange taste sensations

What if My Child Shows These Symptoms?

As mentioned earlier, seek medical attention immediately or call emergency when you notice the first symptoms.

After a medical examination, the doctor may advise therapy or medication for your child. If a kid is facing difficulty closing their eyelid, the doctor may suggest appropriate eye drops.

Children with Bell's palsy may also have difficulty speaking and trouble showing facial expressions. Make sure that the child is receiving sufficient care to cope with these issues. Look for specialist advice from related health professionals.

Bell's palsy has an adverse impact on the child's confidence. Young sufferers experience low self-esteem, become introverted and avoid seeing people. You could invite your child's friends to your home. This will also help expand your child's social circle and give them more confidence to interact with others.

You should remain very patient with your child who might become obsessed with his/her face, asking you repeatedly if their face shows any signs of improvement. It is vital that you explain to your child that they will most likely completely recover from Bell's palsy within a few months.

Remember, be supportive and don't let your child feel different. A child will not appreciate people feeling sorry for him/her as this will make them feel inferior.

School going children have a difficult time coping with Bell's palsy since some children will pick on them and start teasing them about their condition. They could get bullied at school which can be a heartbreaking experience.

Explain to your child how to approach and answer questions about their condition. Children can be vulnerable to bullies, so you can contact your child's teacher and tell him or her about the condition so that they keep an eye out.

Teachers usually accommodate children with Bell's palsy, and they can help the affected child feel comfortable in the classroom. It is necessary to speak to the child's school to be certain they are sensitive to the kid's needs and differences.

As parents, there are certain things you need to be careful about.

1) Kids recover quickly from Bell's palsy. For some children, it may take only a couple of weeks to recover completely. They might experience none of the emotional suffering or pain grownups do.

2) However, some children take longer to get well and may need other treatments such as medicine, therapy, or even surgery. Hence, parents should assess the condition and ask the doctor to decide whether the child is ready to go to school or if he/she needs time to heal and take a break.

3) If a child goes to school, it is vital to inform the teacher that the child might get tired and that his/her eye needs to be

protected. An eye patch is essential to prevent dirt and debris from getting into the eye. If a child wants to go swimming, you need to get some good quality swimming goggles. It is best to let your child do whatever they want, just make sure you have all your bases covered in terms of protecting them both physically and emotionally.

4) Going out in the sun is problematic for children suffering from Bell's palsy since it's difficult to shut the affected eye. Remind the child to wear sunglasses to protect their eye. Sunglasses are also necessary for windy days. Make sure you apply eye drops to your child's eye several times throughout the day. It is also advisable to use an eye patch while the child sleeps. This helps keep the eye moist.

5) Some children experience pain in the face. A moist warm washcloth applied to the affected side of the face may assist in reducing the pain. You should also encourage your child to practice facial exercise as advised by your doctor. It helps speed up recovery.

Bell's palsy: Problems Faced by Teenagers

The teen years are an important part in any individual's life. For some it is time for self-discovery, for others it could be a time of disorientation. Coping with Bell's palsy on the path to adulthood can be a testing time for teenagers. They may face problems such as:

1) Feelings of Low Self-Worth

Teenagers with Bell's palsy suffer from low self-esteem. Feeling incapable to express amusement without being stared at by others affects their confidence. They feel uncomfortable meeting new people. They tend to remain socially distant because they believe they will be unable to interact with people normally.

2) Feeling of Being Alone

Bell's palsy is a rare illness. It affects 1 in 5,000 people each year. As a teenager with Bell's palsy, they feel they are different from everyone else. It may be possible that they may be the only teenagers in their surroundings with Bell's palsy. This creates an overwhelming feeling of being alone. They feel that even their friends and family do not realize what they are going through.

3) **Sense of Poor Body Image**

It's common for teenagers to look at their peers and compare their own appearance. Differences in facial appearance caused by Bell's palsy can have a very powerful impact on a teenager because they become self-conscious and are embarrassed about the way they look.

4) **Feelings of Depression and Grief**

Dealing with feelings of a negative body image and low self-worth can lead to the point of depression among teenagers. A teenager who has suddenly developed Bell's palsy might have a sense of grief take over. They feel that they could have looked so attractive if this condition had not developed.

Furthermore, since 'selfies' and photographs have become such an integral part in a teenager's life, those affected with Bell's palsy feel uncomfortable when being included in pictures. Whether it be a homecoming dance or a prom, teenagers with Bell's palsy may avoid large gatherings because they feel like they will be made fun of or stared at.

5) **Become Withdrawn and Exceedingly Cautious to Express Their Feelings**

Finding it difficult to express feelings of joy freely can be devastating for a teenager. They try to hide their face while smiling or talking. They become socially introverted and less outgoing. The only reason being – they don't want others to notice their collapsed face.

Bell's palsy can affect day to day life aspects; eating, interacting and communicating. Teenagers become self-conscious and avoid outings and dining out with friends and family thinking people might be looking at them.

How to Help People with Bell's Palsy

Since I had facial paralysis at a young age, people around me were used to what I looked like. Not everyone had harsh things to say about my appearance, but clearly, even the 'most concerned friends' were unaware of the full psychological impact Bell's palsy had on me.

Others may not necessarily know how to act or react around people with Bell's palsy.

Raising awareness about the condition is vital. Before helping a loved one with Bell's palsy, it is important to understand what the condition is, how it is caused, and how it psychologically affects an individual. That's why I have written this book!

Imagine you wake up one morning to find that you've developed facial paralysis. For a teenager or young adult who is taking their first step into a new career, college, or entering a new group of friends, this experience is devastating. Instead of socializing more or exploring new opportunities in life, teenagers and young adults who develop Bell's palsy hide from their peers.

Sadly, children, teenagers and even young adults have problems "getting over it and moving on". The grief can be short-term or long-term depending on the severity of the condition. I can understand the feelings of helplessness and sadness at particular moments such as family or other social gatherings.

A great way to support your child could be acknowledging their pain and then presenting your thoughts on how to reduce it. Remember, those suffering from Bell's palsy need emotional support more than any other therapeutic option. We shall be looking at this in particular in our last section, "Providing Moral Support to Patients with Bell's Palsy."

As a friend, it is important that we talk to these teenagers the same way we did before they had the condition. This lets them recognize that our feelings and values for them haven't changed. They are the same person they were before the illness. The worst thing you can do is feel sorry for them. This will not only shatter their confidence but also make them feel inferior.

Educate yourself about the emotional issues that children and teenagers with Bell's palsy face. This will help you provide strong and effective emotional support.

It's always a nice idea to network with parents whose kids have Bell's palsy. You may also surf the internet or look in your local community to find support groups. Through this, teenagers can share their feelings and problems with people who are in a similar position. It will help them recognize that they are not alone dealing with this condition. Also, meeting someone who can relate to their problems can truly enhance their self-esteem.

Chapter Four: Bell's Palsy during Pregnancy

Expecting mothers develop Bell's palsy more frequently, and the reasons are not completely understood. It has been observed that the risk is highest during the third trimester and several weeks after delivery. Luckily, the prognosis for expecting moms is generally good. If a woman is affected with Bell's palsy during pregnancy, there is no effect on the developing fetus.

The symptoms among expecting mothers are the same as described earlier in this book.

Treating Bell's Palsy during Pregnancy

We will look at the treatment methods in more detail later in this book, but for now, let's take a quick look at how Bell's palsy can be treated during pregnancy. You can address symptoms such as pain with pain killers; however, steroids and popular antiviral medication are not recommended.

How Long Will It Take for the Symptoms to Go Away Completely?

Well, you will notice a gradual improvement, but recovery times can vary depending on the extent of nerve damage. Most pregnant women who develop Bell's palsy recover completely in less than six months. In some cases, the recovery time may be longer – this often happens if the patient develops complete facial paralysis.

Pregnant women who develop Bell's palsy are monitored closely for changes in blood pressure. This is because expecting moms suffering from Bell's palsy are also at an increased risk of developing preeclampsia.

Preeclampsia is a serious complication in pregnant women and is characterized by high blood pressure. The increase in blood pressure can cause tremendous damage to vital organs, particularly the kidneys. Preeclampsia is usually spotted after 20 weeks of pregnancy. It can even happen in women who had normal blood pressure during the early weeks of pregnancy.

If left untreated, preeclampsia might lead to serious complications for both the mother and the baby. This condition only has one cure – delivering the baby. That being said; the pregnancy obviously has to be in its final stage for the delivery to take place.

You can talk to your doctor to find out more about preeclampsia. Be sure to monitor your condition and your baby's condition closely to ensure a safe and happy delivery.

Can My Baby Be Affected during Delivery?

Trauma during birth is one of the leading causes of Bell's palsy in children; however, the condition cannot be transferred. Simply put, if you suffer from Bell's palsy during pregnancy, your baby will not be born with it.

Physical injury to the facial nerve can result during 'assisted' delivery. If your baby needs help to move out of the birth canal, your doctor may recommend forceps delivery. The curved ends of the instrument are generally harmless, but in rare cases, they may exert excessive pressure on the baby's head. Any type of compression to the 7th cranial nerve, as you know, can result in the weakness of facial muscles.

In most cases, injury caused by forceps is temporary, and symptoms of facial paralysis go away within a few months. But there have been cases in which the facial paralysis persists for a longer duration.

Bell's palsy due to birth trauma is usually diagnosed by a healthcare provider while the baby is in the hospital. Mild cases, such as those involving just the lower lips may be noticed after a few days. If you suspect facial weakness or notice little or no movement on one side of your baby's face, make an appointment with your baby's pediatrician immediately.

The doctor will carry out a physical examination to determine the exact reason for facial muscle weakness. Further diagnostic tests might be carried out to rule out other common causes of facial palsy such as congenital birth defect, infections and tumor.

Because symptoms caused by birth trauma generally improve on their own within a few months, a team of medical specialists will closely monitor your baby to decide whether medical intervention is needed or not.

Is Bell's Palsy Hereditary?

Presently, there is no strong medical evidence suggesting that Bell's palsy is hereditary, however research is still underway.

Chapter Five: Complications and Myths about Bell's Palsy

Clearing Myths about Bell's Palsy

Just like with any other disease, there are countless myths surrounding Bell's palsy. Here, we've cleared three of the most common myths about this condition. Remember, it's important that we clear up inaccuracies about Bell's palsy to make a better effort at understanding the problem and helping others learn about it.

Bell's palsy Myth #1

Every case of facial paralysis must be Bell's palsy

Fact:

If you recall the section on Bell's palsy causes and symptoms, we've seen that many other conditions such as stroke, tumor, Lyme disease and congenital birth defects can also cause facial paralysis.

So the doctor will tell the patient they have Bell's palsy when facial paralysis or muscle weakness occurs because of an unknown cause.

Bell's palsy Myth #2

Influenza immunization can trigger Bell's palsy

Fact:

There is no scientific evidence that the flu vaccine triggers Bell's palsy. However, some individuals claim that Bell's palsy was caused after flu vaccination in their case. Medical experts suggest that flu vaccination might trigger antibodies that attack normal cells. The 7th cranial nerve may also be affected, which then causes facial paralysis. Research is underway to see if this is actually the cause.

Bell's palsy Myth #3

All Bell's palsy patients are infected by the herpes simplex virus.

Fact:

While medical experts are unable to identify the real cause(s) of Bell's palsy, the herpes simplex virus is still rated as one of the prime suspects. The virus is known to cause swelling and inflammation of the 7th cranial nerve; however, not all Bell's palsy patients have the herpes simplex virus. It is important that healthcare providers conduct a comprehensive diagnosis before starting any treatment method.

Complications of Bell's palsy

Only two in ten patients experience long-term problems and complications resulting from Bell's palsy. Once again, complications that might occur depend on the extent of damage to the 7th cranial nerve.

The most likely complications of Bell's palsy include:

1. **Contracture**

This is a condition where your facial muscles are permanently tense. Contracture can lead to facial scarring – the eye may become smaller, and cheeks may become bulky on the affected side.

2. **Reduced or complete loss of taste**

This is more likely to happen if the 7th cranial nerve doesn't repair properly.

3. **Slurred speech or difficulty speaking**

This complication mainly occurs due to damage to facial muscles.

4. **Eye-mouth synkinesis**

Your eye may wink involuntarily, especially when you are smiling, laughing or eating. This winking can become so sudden and severe that your eye can close completely.

5. Drying of the eye and corneal ulceration

Corneal ulceration is likely to happen when the thin protective tear film in the eye becomes less effective. An ulcer is more commonly seen if the patient is unable to shut their eye completely. Dry eyes occur as a result of reduced tear production. Both corneal ulceration and dry eyes may lead to further eye infections.

6. Excessive tear production

Some people experience excessive tear production. Tearing is initiated spontaneously while eating and laughing and is also known as 'crocodile tears.'

7. Ramsay Hunt syndrome

If Bell's palsy is caused by the varicella-zoster virus, there is a possibility that patients may develop Ramsay Hunt syndrome. This condition is extremely rare, and only less than 2% of patients with Bell's palsy are at risk of being affected. Ramsay Hunt syndrome is characterized by the presence of blisters on the tongue and inside the ears. The condition generally responds to steroids and antiviral medication.

Long-term complications of Bell's palsy are more likely if:

a. You suffer from complete paralysis, i.e. there is no movement on either side of your face.

b. Your facial nerve is badly damaged.

c. You have diabetes and hypertension (high blood pressure).

d. You are over 60 years of age.

e. You are pregnant.

f. You show no signs of recovery even after six weeks.

Facial Palsy and Synkinesis

What is Synkinesis?

Synkinesis is said to occur when your facial muscles move unwantedly. The condition is very common in people who are recovering from prolonged facial palsy.

What Really Happens?

Technically, the term synkinesis means simultaneous movement and is a result of abnormal facial nerve regeneration. Certain facial muscles contract with the 'working' muscles, which leads to uncontrollable expressions.

Unfortunately, the 7th cranial nerve is poorly insulated during the recovery phase. Healthy and uninjured nerves, on the other hand, are properly insulated by a thin layer of specialized 'fat' cells called the myelin sheath.

Since the facial nerve has faulty insulation, messages specifically intended for one particular set of muscles are also picked up by another muscle. This is what results in the movement of more than one muscle at the same time. For example, your eye might close when you try to smile. Even though these movements are temporary, they sadly tend to become a habit. Some people continue to show 'linked movements' even after they recover from Bell's palsy.

What Are the Causes?

Your body's natural healing mechanism is also partially responsible for these unwanted movements. Simply put, the recovering nerve fibers are implanted into different unwanted muscle groups that produce the undesirable simultaneous facial responses.

Synkinesis can also happen when the facial nerve is reconnected to a wrong group of facial muscles after surgery. Most surgical treatment options for Bell's and facial palsy involve cutting the 7th cranial nerve and sewing it with a healthy group of facial muscles. Sometimes, when the nerve fibers are reattached to the muscles, they connect to the wrong group of facial muscles causing abnormal facial movement.

Surprisingly, the muscles in your face tend to work together while facial nerves are recovering. The different groups of muscles join forces to help accomplish a task such as smiling or blinking an eye. Because all muscle groups are working together, it is hard to coordinate specific facial movements.

Your facial muscles also fail to follow the assigned sequence of activity; hence small movements happen as one 'large' movement which obviously doesn't look natural. Muscles affected by facial palsy also forget which movement should happen first and start competing with the good muscles. Sometimes the affected muscles are overworked in this 'tug of war' resulting in short, stiff muscle fibers.

Synkinesis: Basics You Need to Know

1. Symptoms of synkinesis only show on the side of the face affected by Bell's palsy.
2. Facial palsy patients notice symptoms largely in the cheek, chin, and eye and neck area.
3. Even the mild symptoms appear more prominent when the good side is compared to the affected side of the face.

The Look and Feel

The condition may show up in different ways. The most common observations include:

1. The eye squints whenever you smile.
2. Your cheek might rise as you try to close your eyes.
3. Your neck feels tight when you try to whistle.
4. Facial twitching, especially in the neck and chin area becomes more common.

5. Facial muscles typically in the forehead and eyebrow area become tight, causing discomfort. You may find it difficult to move tight and stiff muscles.
6. Even when the affected side of the face is relaxed, the mouth appears to be pulled up. Your cheek may appear bulky, and the eyes might squint.

What are the Common Symptoms of Synkinesis?

Most patients who develop synkinesis believe that their muscles are weak, especially if they become too tight. Following are the characteristic symptoms you would notice during synkinesis.

Facial muscles on the affected side become tighter than the muscles on the good side.

This simply means that the facial muscles on the affected side have a higher tone. The muscles can work twice or three times more than the good muscles as you try to move them. This is one of the reasons your mouth is pulled upwards, and cheeks appear bulky even when you are resting.

Continuous overwork might cause your facial muscles to become short and tight.

Overworked muscles are under constant stress and become extremely difficult to move. Patients with synkinesis cannot move and control the facial muscles correctly when they want to express themselves.

Can You Predict Synkinesis?

Will you always feel some kind of tightening or pain in your facial muscles? Well, synkinesis is somewhat predictable; however, the severity of the symptoms can differ greatly among patients.

Before we discuss the predictable pattern, let us first differentiate between true paralysis (weak muscles) and synkinesis. For this quick test, all you need to do is stand in front of a mirror. What do you see? If your facial tone is normal and you can observe noticeable movements, the abnormal movements are a result of facial synkinesis.

Most patients recovering from facial palsy and Bell's palsy experience eye closure, in particular, when they try to smile. Sometimes, the eyelids tend to twitch or close suddenly while the patient is trying to laugh.

Synkinesis also affects patients who have reacquired their facial tone. The patients are unable to pull the affected corner of the mouth upwards when they smile – people assume that their mouth is not moving due to muscle weakness, i.e. loss of muscle tone. The reason, on the other hand, is synkinesis or simultaneous movement, not facial paralysis.

The inability to move corners of the mouth is obvious because muscles that droop towards the corner of mouth, i.e. zygomaticus major and minor, work simultaneously with depressor anguli oris, platysma, and mentalis, i.e. muscles responsible to elevate the corner of your mouth.

Other characteristic patterns of synkinesis include narrowing of the eyes and increased muscle tone (tightness, spasm and contracture) in the chin. In addition to abnormal movement patterns around the eyes, chin and mouth, synkinesis also causes the affected cheek to become tight and bulky.

What Are Your Treatment Options?

Three popular methods namely physical therapy, Botox injections (botulinum toxin) and surgery are employed by doctors to treat synkinesis. The choice of treatment method depends on the severity of the symptoms. Your doctor can start the treatment any time after synkinesis has occurred. Interestingly, successful treatment of synkinesis is possible even if therapy is started years after the patient has suffered Bell's or facial palsy.

Physical Therapy – Neuromuscular Retraining

Physical therapy for the treatment of synkinesis is very different from the therapy utilized for other medical complications such as lower back pain and arthritis. Facial physical therapy or neuromuscular retraining during synkinesis is very similar to learning to sing with a hoarse voice.

Any singer with a hoarse voice will learn to adjust their vocal cords to overcome poor sound. Similarly, patients with Bell's palsy or facial palsy focus on coordinating different muscles to achieve controlled, synchronized and natural looking facial muscle movements. This physical therapy is extremely useful in overcoming the activity of unwanted muscles.

More information on physical therapy can be found under the treatment section, but here's a quick overview to help you understand synkinesis better.

Your healthcare provider will refer you to a qualified therapist who will then identify the muscles that show linked movements or are contracting abnormally. Facial muscles that fail to follow the 'natural sequence' of activity are also identified.

Small and simple exercises, usually, are then suggested in order to retrain your muscles at the neurologic level. Facial and neck muscles on the affected side are massaged and stretched, however patients are advised not apply excessive force. Remember, you have to re-train overactive, stiff muscles so that your facial muscles become coordinated, and this might take some time. Almost 90% of the physical therapy involves personalized exercises that can be done at home. You can always refer to your healthcare provider if you have specific questions related to physical therapy.

Botox Injections

The second most popular therapy for synkinesis is the use of Botox or (botulinum toxin-A) injections. Your therapist may use Botox in combination with facial physical therapy in some cases.

Botox injections work by calming down overactive muscles. Overworked muscles in the eyes (orbicularis), neck (platysma), and chin (mentalis) are usually targeted. Your therapist will inject the botulinum toxin in the tight areas to restore facial symmetry. Often, healthcare providers also use Botox on the normal side of the face (forehead, lower lips and corners of the eye) to make the face symmetrical.

Surgical Treatment

Surgical treatment of synkinesis is only utilized when the other two methods (i.e. physical therapy and Botox) fail to give the desired results.

Selective neurolysis is the latest surgical innovation in the treatment of synkinesis. During this surgery, a certified surgeon will release the platysma muscle and decrease activity of the facial nerves that pull the mouth down. This surgical intervention will allow the corners of the mouth to move upwards again.

Other surgical treatments of synkinesis involve eyelid surgery and facelift. Your doctor is in the best position to determine whether or not you are the right candidate for synkinesis surgery.

Chapter Six: Treating Bell's Palsy – Non-Surgical Options

The treatment used during Bell's palsy depends on the cause and severity of the symptoms. It can range from simple lubricating eye drops and steroid medication to eyelid weights for people having difficulty closing their eye. A combination of anti-viral medication and oral steroids is known to improve the chances of recovery among Bell's palsy patients.

Even without any formal treatment, a lot of people completely recover from Bell's palsy. Nonetheless, there are various therapeutic options that help reduce the risk of complications. There is a dispute among researchers about the most effective cure for Bell's palsy. But most doctors use a combination of antiviral medications and steroids for the treatment.

Oral Medication

Prednisolone

The primary concern in the management of Bell's palsy is to remove the origin of the injury to the facial nerve without delay. In this regard, Prednisolone is found to be very effective as stated by numerous studies. This is a prescription drug often used to treat inflammation and swelling. You may have seen it used in medication such as Orapred, Millipred, Omnipred, Econopred, or Flo-Pred. As time goes on, damage to the nerve can increase. Thus, it is advisable to use steroids within 72 hours of the symptoms appearing.

Early treatment with Prednisolone helps reduce inflammation, thereby improving the chances of complete recovery from Bell's palsy. Prednisolone is typically prescribed for a 10-day course in which patients generally take two tablets a day.

Pregnant women and mothers who are breastfeeding are advised to consult their doctor before taking Prednisolone. Not all who take steroids have side effects. However, some patients may experience mood swings, depression and anxiety. Consult your doctor immediately if you experience any of the following side effects:

a. Headache
b. Indigestion
c. Dizziness
d. Increased appetite
e. Nausea
f. Oral thrush
g. Loss of sleep

Prednisolone is available in tablet, liquid and concentrated form that can be taken orally. It is recommended that you take Prednisone with food as advised by your doctor.

Often, patients are prescribed to take Prednisone one to four times a day. Your personal dosage will depend on the severity of the symptoms and how well you respond to the treatment.

Precautions to Remember

1. Follow the directions carefully when taking Prednisone and do not change the dosage. Remember, you cannot take more or less steroid medication to speed up recovery. If your doctor prescribes a concentrated solution of Prednisone, it may be taken with liquid.

2. Do inform your doctor if you are taking grapefruit or grapefruit juice because it may cause a negative reaction when consumed with Prednisone. Another thing you need to remember is that your dose of Prednisone can be changed during the treatment.

3. Never stop taking steroid medication without informing your doctor. Remember, if you stop taking Prednisone

suddenly, your body may not have enough natural 'defense' substances to function normally.

4. Abrupt withdrawal of steroid medication might produce symptoms such as fatigue, weight loss, mouth sores, changes in skin color and upset stomach. If you experience any of these symptoms, contact your doctor immediately.

5. Steroid medication is known to decrease your ability to fight infections, so make sure you stay away from people who are sick during the course of your therapy. Try to wash your hands often. Be sure you avoid people who are suffering from chickenpox and measles.

6. You might be instructed to follow a diet rich in potassium and calcium while taking Prednisone. Your doctor may also ask you to reduce your salt intake. If needed, you might be asked to take a calcium or potassium supplement along with Prednisone.

Antiviral Drugs

As viral infections have a role in the etiology of Bell's palsy, antiviral drugs are also used to treat the condition. Although antiviral drugs, if taken alone, have no impact on recovery, they are used in combination with Prednisolone for greater effectiveness.

Acyclovir (Zovirax) and valacyclovir (Valtrex) are sometimes used to treat Bell's palsy. They are known to prevent the development of infection if a virus is identified to have caused the inflammation of the facial nerve. It is worth mentioning that this treatment is offered only if the condition is severe.

Treatment with Botulinum Toxin

There are a number of neurotransmitters (special chemical substances) inside your body that control the transmission of electrical signals. Acetylcholine is the neurotransmitter responsible for transmitting electrical messages that help facial muscles contract.

Facial paralysis caused by Bell's palsy is sudden; however, you never know how long these effects may last. Botulinum toxin or simply Botox injections help paralyzed muscles relax and restore facial symmetry. Botulinum toxin is a protein produced by bacterium Clostridium botulinum and this toxin blocks the release of acetylcholine.

Your doctor will inject the toxin into affected muscles on the paralyzed side, causing them to relax as I mentioned earlier in the treatment of synkinesis section. The result is a more symmetrical face. A very fine needle is used during the procedure; therefore, you will experience very little pain.

Sometimes, Botox injections are also used on the normal side of the face to restore symmetry. What you need to remember is that Botox is a temporary solution and results may vary with each individual. You may have to repeat the treatment if the symptoms don't subside. Your doctor will be in a better position to guide you about this.

Physical Therapy

Physical therapy such as biofeedback, facial exercises, thermotherapy and massages are used to speed up recovery from Bell's palsy. Not only does it prevent facial drooping from occurring again, but it also helps facial muscles regain their strength.

After a thorough physical examination, a physical therapist identifies the weaknesses caused by this condition.

Physical therapy helps patients perform daily activities since it retrains muscles into working the way you want them to work. Physical therapy is intended to help people relearn their facial movements and is commonly referred to as initiation exercises.

Once patients have successfully overcome the challenging period of relearning, physical therapy is used to make muscles 'relearn' certain movements. Exercise strengthens facial muscles so that they can perform the same functions as they were able to before the onset of Bell's Palsy.

Cognitive Behavior Therapy (CBT)

Cognitive Behavior Therapy (CBT) is a type of emotional therapy used to treat a wide range of issues. Teenagers and adults suffering from Bell's palsy can receive psychological therapy to overcome their emotional difficulties.

Bell's palsy, as you can guess, limits a person's positive thoughts and slowly replaces them with negative emotions. Young adults in particular feel depressed and miserable in this challenging situation. CBT helps Bell's palsy sufferers respond more positively to the situation. The therapist talks to you and explains how your thoughts are affected by what you think and feel. Simply put, you will learn how negative thoughts and assumptions can be converted into more positive ones.

What you need to remember is that cognitive behavior therapy is not an instant solution or fix. It may take some time before a Bell's palsy patient can look at their situation from a positive, fresh perspective.

Patients with Bell's palsy find it difficult to think (cognitive) and act (behavioral) the same way they used to before being affected. However, events occurring in the present are far more important than what has taken place in the past. There is substantial evidence that CBT helps people overcome depression, anxiety, low self-esteem and negative thoughts.

Bell's palsy sufferers often feel anxious while interacting with others and experience constant depressing thoughts. They are reluctant to meet new people, and this behavior is seen in almost every patient, no matter what the cause. Some patients just want to hide so that they no longer have to face anyone. What's really upsetting is the fact that this emotional trauma is severe in teenagers and young adults.

Because of the impact Bell's palsy has on a person's appearance, the best course of action would be to see how patients feel about themselves. Remember, dealing with emotional elements is as important as treating physical symptoms. CBT can be implemented more successfully if the therapist is well aware of the patient's behavior, thoughts and feelings.

What Happens during Cognitive Behavioral Therapy?

A certified therapist will first decide whether or not CBT will be useful in your case. Your first assessment session will most likely identify your feelings and thoughts about having Bell's palsy. CBT sessions are usually between six and twelve weeks.

The first step, as mentioned earlier, is to identify your feelings and thoughts. Your therapist will then help you break them into smaller parts so you can easily evaluate how these emotions are affecting you.

Analyzing CBT Sessions

CBT involves five different aspects, namely; situation, thoughts, emotions, actions and physical feelings.

Situation as you can guess is the problem or event that you are facing. If you are facing any difficult situation, your brain is bombarded with emotions, thoughts and feelings, all of which compel you to take action. This action is how you respond. It can be helpful or unhelpful.

For example:

You enter a place where not many people know you. Suddenly, everyone starts looking at your face. At this point, you can have two types of thoughts.

Unhelpful: People only see my facial disfigurement.

Helpful: They are looking to see if they know me.

When your thoughts are unhelpful, the most obvious emotions will be sadness, anger and frustration. You will want to go home and avoid further interaction with new people.

On the other hand, if you have helpful thoughts in your head, you will be excited to find out whose present at the place you have just arrived at. Since you will be feeling confident, there will be no hesitation in introducing yourself and finding out if anyone knows you.

Can you see the difference your thoughts can have on your responses? Remember, the more effort you put into identifying your positive feelings, the easier it will be to cope with Bell's palsy.

Your cognitive behavioral therapist will advise you to maintain a diary. Whenever you feel depressed, write down the situation and thoughts and explore them with your therapist in the next CBT session.

Unfortunately, many people with Bell's palsy assume that others find them unattractive. This is one of the reasons Bell's palsy patients have problems combating negative thoughts and ideas. Try to think positively as this will help you manage different feelings and situations with a great deal of ease.

Electrical Stimulation

Electrical stimulation is also a popular technique used to treat Bell's palsy. When you smile, raise your eyebrow or simply close your eyes, your 7th facial nerve is at work.

Patients with Bell's palsy may experience difficulties such as the inability to express emotion on the affected side of the face. There are problems closing the eyes, and the mouth may collapse on one side. The facial nerve in Bell's palsy either gets inflamed or compressed due to the condition. That is why the electrical impulses fail to travel along the damaged facial nerve to reach the muscles that need to move.

The ineffective communication between the brain and facial muscles causes the muscles to become droopy and weak. Electrical stimulation aims at imitating the function of electrical impulses through the use of a mild current. This passage of current is thought to assist the restoration of nerve function and overall muscle tone.

Electrical stimulation should be carried out under the supervision of a specialist. Without the guidance of an expert, patients are advised not to attempt it in any case. The technique may cause problems if it is carried out without adequate supervision.

It's important to keep in mind that the facial nerve is capable of recovering naturally. Therefore, therapists and medical experts give time for the nerve to heal without any intervention. Meanwhile, patients are encouraged to carry out facial massages tenderly that will assist blood circulation and maintain muscle health. At the start of the recovery phase, patients must try to focus more on massaging their face and protecting their eye. They can gently massage their face in a circular motion by using their fingers.

Once the facial nerve starts recovering, it begins to emit electrical signals in the facial muscles.

If the facial muscles are unable to regain their natural tone, patients can go ahead with electrical stimulation after consulting a certified healthcare professional.

As mentioned earlier, the technique has to be carried out very carefully. Failure to do so can result in overstimulation of the muscles. This can be a painful experience for patients since muscles become stiff and can twitch uncontrollably.

Electrical stimulation helps improve the contraction of muscles, which helps achieve facial symmetry.

Biofeedback Therapy

Facial paralysis, at some point, causes a disruption in nerve signals sent to the facial muscles. When this confusion continues to exist, there are interruptions in the feedback sent to the brain about the affected side of the face. Since your mind is always busy, it ultimately forgets about the lack of communication on the affected side of the face. It only relies on the good side and you may notice that the facial muscles that remain unaffected slowly begin to dominate.

What Is Biofeedback?

Bell's palsy rehabilitation via biofeedback is all about getting your entire face back into action, but you need a little help from outside.

Biofeedback is a method through which people can learn to control their body's functions. Biofeedback involves using sensors placed strategically over the human body. These sensors help receive feedback about the body, hence, the term biofeedback. This feedback assists people in making minor changes to their body over time, such as relaxing specific muscles to reduce the intensity of pain. In short, biofeedback allows you to use your thoughts to control certain aspects of your body, such as muscles.

During recovery, Bell's palsy patients reach a stage where their face feels incredibly tight. The eye may shut without any indication while eating or talking. Some patients also feel that they are making funny faces when smiling. It is the faulty communication system between your face and brain that is letting you down. Biofeedback allows you to learn how to control muscles to display the expression you want.

What Are the Different Types of Biofeedback?

There are three most commonly used forms of biofeedback therapy including:

1. Electromyography (EMG) used to measure muscle tension.

2. Thermal biofeedback used to measure skin temperature.

3. Electroencephalography (EEG) or neuro-feedback used to measure brain wave activity.

What Happens during Biofeedback Therapy?

A typical biofeedback session will involve attaching tiny electrodes to your skin. These electrodes then send information to a small box that translates the signals your body is giving out. You will see lines that vary in pitch on a computer screen. The biofeedback therapist in charge will then guide you through some mental exercises. Soon, with trial and error, you will learn exercises that can bring about the activity you want on the affected side of your face.

You will also be taught relaxation techniques and exercises that need to be done at home for at least 5 - 10 minutes every day.

Are There Any Risks Associated with Biofeedback Sessions?

Each biofeedback session usually lasts less than 60 minutes. The number of sessions you require depends on the severity of the condition.

This therapy is considered safe. No side effects have been reported to date. What's even better is that you don't need any special preparation for the treatment.

If you're looking to find a qualified biofeedback therapist, start by asking your healthcare provider or another healthcare professional. Your doctor is in a better position to recommend someone who has experience in the same area.

Will My Movements Be Natural?

Some people worry if they will ever be able to portray facial expressions normally again; the same way they were able to before Bell's palsy.

Remember, biofeedback sessions will help you discover ways you can control muscles on the affected side of the face and after some time, you can smile without having to think about it.

Is This Treatment Only for Bell's Palsy?

Of course not! There is massive evidence relating to the use of this technique for other medical conditions and different muscle groups in your body. You can always ask your doctor whether biofeedback is something you should incorporate into your treatment.

Facial Rehabilitation

Facial rehabilitation therapy is another known method used to promote recovery among patients affected by Bell's palsy. It incorporates various methods such as facial exercise; massages and stretching techniques that help people relearn facial movements and develop stronger movement control as well.

Successful treatment and the subsequent choice of therapy for Bell's palsy depends on determining the cause of the condition. Once the diagnosis is confirmed, it is also important to assess the severity of the symptoms and how long you've had this condition before any therapy is started.

An expert of facial rehabilitation will assess your diagnosis and will refer you to a speech or language therapist depending on your symptoms and present situation.

What Will You Experience?

Wondering what happens in this rehabilitation therapy? Here are a few things that you can expect from a specialized therapist:

1) Initial sessions with the therapist will involve the assessment of symptoms and condition. Patients may be asked about their existing symptoms, and they will also be asked what improves or worsens their condition.

2) Medical history can also be reviewed to help the therapist evaluate the patient's condition. From these assessment results, the specialist will be able to develop an individualized plan for therapy.

3) Typically, facial electromyography (EMG) is an essential part in the diagnosis of patients with Bell's palsy. It helps detect the presence of the condition and evaluates the extent of damage to the facial nerve. This also helps the therapist get an idea of the rate of recovery. There is no need to worry about this test. It is a simple, painless procedure and will not take much time.

4) If the therapist doesn't have access to an EMG machine, he or she can evaluate the condition through careful inspection of facial features including the cheeks, lips, brows, etc. The therapist might ask patients to raise their eyebrows, close their eyes or smile widely. Through these actions, the therapist will be able to observe the symmetry and movement of the face. This will also help evaluate nerve functions.

5) After this, the therapist will be able to judge the extent of weakness of the facial muscles. Subsequently, patients will be guided as to how they can protect their face and eyes. Therapists will perform the role of a coach and educate patients about how they can perform their daily life functions with this condition.

6) If patients have severe problems, such as extremely dry eyes or slurred speech, the therapist may refer them to a specialist. An ophthalmologist (a physician who specializes in the surgical or medical care of the eyes) or language therapist would then be able to manage the specific symptoms.

Guidance and Useful Advice

Patients may receive various wellness advice regarding treatment and care. Usually, caregivers offer suggestions and guidance concerning the following issues:

Eye Protection and Care

a. Your therapist will advise you to protect your eye from becoming infected and dry. Artificial tears and eye patches are highly recommended for maximum protection.

b. Patients are also encouraged to blink their eyes. By covering their eyelids with their fingertips, patients can learn to how to imitate blinking. This is particularly important to keep the eye moist and protected from external debris.

Managing Daily-life Activities Such As Eating and Oral Hygiene

Due to the loss of control of the lips and mouth, Bell's palsy makes it difficult for people to eat and drink normally. Patients will be guided to eat in a way that they do not bite their lips or cheeks.

Therapists can also inform patients to pay special attention to their oral health. Bell's palsy affects the production of saliva and decreases sensation on the paralyzed side of the mouth. Therapists suggest regular brushing to ensure good oral hygiene.

Speech Support

Speech may be mildly slurred due to this condition. Patients may receive advice on how to work on this problem. Therapists might suggest various facial exercises to overcome this difficulty.

Customized Home Exercise Plan

After the careful inspection of medical records and facial functions, the rehabilitation therapist will brief the patient about the various treatment options based on the diagnosis and particular symptoms.

1. One of the unique aspects of facial rehabilitation is that each treatment and therapy is designed according to the special needs of the patient. This typically involves an individualized exercise plan that can be carried out at home by patients themselves.

2. The customized home exercise plan aims to promote symmetrical and synchronized facial movement. With regular and consistent implementation of the program, patients exhibit considerable improvement in facial functions. It is a great plan due the fact that it reduces the number of billed clinic hours and increases overall practice hours.

3. In order to enhance the patient's understanding and to keep a track on recovery, therapists can also incorporate photographic and video assessments.

4. Patients are educated regarding their facial anatomy and working of the facial nerve. It is an integral part of the therapy plan. Once patients understand how their face functions, it is easier for them to monitor and keep track of their recovery.

5. Initially, patients are trained to carry out small facial movements. They are advised to use mirrors for help. Remember, therapists don't want to cause muscular fatigue on the affected side of the face. Thus, the exercise sessions are kept short.

6. Once the recovery starts, assisted facial movements become part of the exercise plan. They help patients relearn facial movements and focus on the symmetry of these movements.

7. The side of the face that is affected by Bell's palsy suffers from muscle tightness and patients may experience spasms as well. Therefore, one vital part of this rehabilitation therapy is relaxing these muscles and facial nerve. This involves stretching techniques that help reduce stiffness in the affected facial muscles.

8. Some patients experience abnormal patterns of muscle movement due to Bell's palsy. This condition is referred as synkinesis, which we discussed earlier. The home plan addresses these issues as well and involves massage techniques that don't only prevent muscular spasms, but also reduce these involuntary movements.

Here are a few things that you need to keep in mind:

1. Avoid urgency and do not excessively strain your muscles when performing the home exercise plan designed by your therapist. The facial nerve takes time to heal and

regeneration takes place slowly and gradually, so be gentle. If you try to put in extra effort to move these affected muscles, it may cause abnormal movement patterns.

2. Once you start to regain control of facial movements, visit your therapist to upgrade your home exercise plan. Required adjustments to the plan will be made by the therapist depending on your needs and progress. You may have to be patient throughout this process. Rehabilitation therapy takes time and a lot of commitment. But bear in mind, this is your key to success.

3. Just a friendly reminder – do not cheat. Needless to say, good compliance is crucial in achieving your desired results.

4. Another important thing – practice every day! It is recommended to remain in touch with your therapist via phone or email if you cannot visit in person. This way you can communicate your concerns and queries and the therapist may be able to address them over the phone.

B-Vitamins Therapy

Vitamins are necessary for your body to function properly. The B-vitamins collectively are included under the list of essential 'micronutrients' and are quite useful in converting proteins and carbohydrates into energy. Also, there is a strong link between the B-vitamins, i.e. B-1, B-6, B-12 and cell repair.

You can get B-vitamins by consuming enriched whole grains, dark green vegetables, nuts, and most meat and dairy products. It is a good idea to talk about your specific vitamin B requirements with your healthcare provider before adding any multi-vitamins or supplements to your diet.

A study held at Oregon State University concluded that athletes who lack B-vitamins in their diet are unable to repair damaged cells and muscles at the same pace as their peers who consume a diet rich in vitamin B. Even a minor vitamin B deficiency can result in reduced performance and poor muscle recovery.

Adding B-vitamins to your diet can help speed up recovery and ease the symptoms of facial paralysis.

Vitamin B-12

Vitamin B-12 plays a vital role in the maintenance of various physiological functions. Vitamin B-12 is required for metabolism (the way your body breaks down nutrients to release energy), red blood cell production and the maintenance of the central nervous system. Vitamin B-12's positive effect on the nervous system may play a supportive role in the treatment of Bell's palsy. Simply put, adding a vitamin B-12 supplement to your diet will help boost facial nerve repair and growth.

It's also an option to have vitamin B-12 injections to treat Bell's palsy. These injections are administered directly into the affected side of the face, and are thought to help by stimulating the facial nerve and reducing inflammation, and can speed up recovery

As with any mineral and vitamin supplement, or other type of treatment, consult your doctor prior to adding vitamin B supplements to your diet plan.

Remember

Vitamin B12 not only actively protects nerves, but it also reduces nerve inflammation.

Many people prefer to use natural vitamin B-12 to speed up recovery instead of steroids.

Vitamin B-1

Adding vitamin B-1 to your diet may prove beneficial in reducing the duration of paralysis. It may bring the total recovery time down from 3 to 4 weeks to less than 3 weeks.

Vitamin B-6

Pyridoxine or vitamin B-6 is used by your body to convert food into glucose. This vitamin also plays an important part in making the nervous system run smoothly, and this is why you can use Pyridoxine to help relieve symptoms of Bell's palsy. Studies show that vitamin B-6 can help restore the facial nerve.

What you need to remember is that most supportive care for Bell's palsy is probably sitting in your kitchen or medicine cupboard already.

Acupuncture

Conventional methods of treating Bell's palsy include the use of steroids, physical therapy and surgical procedures. The chances of recovery are increased if you start treating the condition quickly. In addition to the standard procedures, complete restoration of nerve function is also possible with the use of alternative treatment methods. One such treatment is acupuncture.

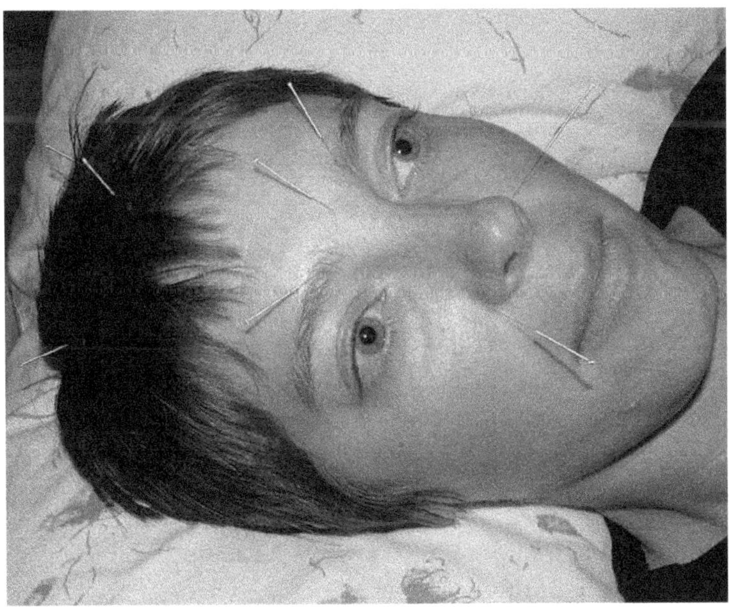

Credit: *'Facial acupuncture' by mscaprikell from Wikipedia Commons (https://commons.wikimedia.org/wiki/File:Facial_acupuncture.jpg) under the Creative Commons Attribution-Share Alike 2.0 Generic*

Recent medical research suggests that acupuncture can help alleviate the symptoms of Bell's palsy. In fact, the practice of acupuncture to treat Bell's palsy is growing in popularity worldwide. Acupuncture is a Chinese medical technique that has been used for generations. It involves the insertion of fine needles into the skin. It is practiced not only to cure diseases or relieve pain, but also to improve general health and well-being. Today, this ancient practice is used to treat a wide variety of health conditions globally.

This Chinese technique is believed to stimulate the central nervous system, which in turn affects the release of useful biochemical substances such as neurotransmitters and hormones. The release of these substances boosts your body's in-built natural healing system and promotes emotional and physical wellbeing.

What Happens in Acupuncture?

Acupuncture is generally recommended twice a week. These sessions help improve the overall facial nerve function and tone of facial muscles among Bell's palsy patients.

As mentioned earlier, a typical acupuncture session will involve inserting very fine needles into your skin at specific points. The primary aim of this practice is to balance the flow of energy in your body.

As these thin needles move through the layers of your skin, they are believed to rebalance the flow of energy inside the body. This condition is sometimes referred to as 'Wind Attack' among the traditional Chinese.

Bell's palsy according to Traditional Chinese medicine is said to develop due to exposure to wind that causes inflammation of the facial nerve. This results in qi or chi (vital energy) deficiency and the disruption of natural blood flow. Qi, also pronounced chi, is translated as life force or natural energy. Therefore, acupuncture sessions specifically target the effect of wind on the body and seek to improve blood circulation to the face and stimulate qi.

For successful recovery, traditional Chinese medicine practitioners recommend a combination of herbs to be used along with routine acupuncture. According to Chinese medicine experts, a weak and deficient immune system is also responsible for the development of Bell's palsy. They believe that if your body has a strong, healthy defense mechanism, your chances of being affected by Bell's palsy are minimal. Therefore, certified acupuncturists also place a strong emphasis on maintaining a healthy lifestyle.

Your acupuncture session with a certified therapist might include numerous tips on staying stress-free and following a nutritious diet plan. Make sure you avoid stress and get an ample amount of rest throughout your acupuncture treatment.

The main reason acupuncture is becoming such a popular option for Bell's palsy treatment is that it has a very holistic approach. Not only will you notice an improvement in your symptoms, but your body's natural healing mechanism is also given a boost. If you are apprehensive about using steroids that might cause certain side effects, then acupuncture is an excellent alternative. However like most treatments, this ancient medicine practice also has a slight possibility of adverse effects.

What Are the Risks?

According to several independent surveys, acupuncture is found to be harmless; however, it is always advised that you visit a qualified, reputable practitioner. The risk of serious side effects in acupuncture is minimal – it is seen to be less than 1 in 10,000.

Still, 8-12% of patients undergoing treatment may experience some minor side effects such as:

1. Drowsiness or tiredness

This is a typical reaction after acupuncture and should not be a matter of great concern. Your body needs rest in order to boost its natural healing mechanism, so make sure you're getting enough sleep.

2. Feeling soreness and pain where needles are inserted in the skin

You may feel sore at specific points where the needles are inserted, but this pain normally dispels in less than 24 hours.

3. Bleeding or bruising

The majority of patients don't experience these symptoms. In some cases, bruising or bleeding might occur on the area being treated.

4. Fainting

For anxious patients or those afraid of needles, certain side effects such as fainting and vomiting can become a concern. It can be a physically intense process for faint-hearted patients, so make sure you consult your therapist for further advice.

5. Other risks

Serious risks such as infections and tissue damage are particularly uncommon. A professionally trained practitioner uses only disposable needles for the treatment and is well-versed in anatomy. Please do not hesitate in discussing safety issues with your acupuncturist before you begin treatment.

Is Acupuncture Right for Me?

People who have bleeding disorders such as hemophilia should avoid acupuncture. This is because there can be a possible danger of bleeding from the area the needle was inserted. This also applies to patients who are taking anticoagulants for blood thinning. These medications prevent blood from clotting. So before having an acupuncture treatment, do not forget to seek advice from your doctor if you have any such disorders.

Pregnant women should also seek the advice of their doctor before beginning acupuncture treatment. In general, acupuncture is highly effective during pregnancy because it reduces pain.

People with pacemakers must avoid electro-acupuncture. Acupuncture has different variations, and it's not always about the insertion of needles. Some treatments require electrical stimulation. So for patients who have pacemakers, this could be bothersome or extremely harmful as it may disrupt the function of the device.

If you have metal allergies, especially to stainless steel, acupuncture may not be a good option for you. Moreover, patients with unstable diabetes and immune disorders must seek expert advice before having acupuncture.

Speech Therapy

Some people experience speech problems due to Bell's palsy. This is because the facial nerve has the responsibility of keeping facial muscles toned and is responsible for lip movements required for clear speech. So because of the malfunction of the facial nerve in Bell's palsy, patients experience either partial or complete facial weakness.

Those affected with Bell's palsy may find it hard to pronounce certain words correctly, especially those with the letters B and P. However, the trouble in talking typically depends on the severity of muscle weakness.

Patients become reluctant to talk to other people and become very embarrassed due to their slurred speech. This is particularly awkward for school-going children who develop Bell's palsy. Sadly, they can turn out to be an easy target for bullying and teasing at school.

In addition, patients whose careers require talking to others or giving presentations have to deal with several challenges. Because of slurred speech, they may become self-conscious, which may affect the quality of their work. This is typically true for professions such as acting, teaching, training or sales.

As I've mentioned throughout the book, you should not worry. The majority of people affected with Bell's palsy show no signs of slurred speech once they recover completely. Here are some simple tips that are particularly significant in dealing with speech difficulties:

1. Keep your head held high while talking. One of the best tips to speak in a better manner is to keep your head held high while talking. For instance, if you have to speak in class, don't tuck your chin downwards into your chest. Always project your voice by looking straight in front of you. This will help you sound clear.

2. Keep your conversation short. Weariness and fatigue can also aggravate speech problems in people suffering from Bell's palsy. In this situation; you may consider cutting your sentences and conversation a bit short. You may use gestures, eye contact and other facial expressions to help you communicate efficiently.

3. If you are trying to speak in a hurry, it will in no way help your cause. Always slow down and take your time. Pause-frequently, speak slowly and don't get stressed. Try to use small sentences to convey your message. Others will find it easier to comprehend what you are saying.

Other Helpful Suggestions

1. If you have to give a presentation or talk to clients who aren't aware of your speech problem, you may let them know beforehand. It is also a good idea to ask for feedback from your listeners. For example, you can ask them whether they understand you or not.

2. Since dry mouth can also be a problem with Bell's palsy, it is advised to take frequent sips of water throughout the conversation. If you have an excessively dry mouth, you may consider using saliva stimulants or artificial saliva that can help moisten the mouth. Your healthcare provider can provide more information about this.

3. It is always recommended to face the audience while speaking. This enables them to read your lips and

understand what you are saying. Also try to reduce any distractions in the surrounding area while you speak. For instance, you may turn off the television or other background sounds so that listeners can hear you without any trouble.

Speech Therapy for Children

Children who are born with Bell's palsy have to experience greater difficulty when it comes to slurred speech. They require specialized help such as coaching from a certified speech and language therapist as early as possible.

After some basic diagnosis and assessment, therapists will be able to advise you on management and support for speech problems your child experiences. In many cases, qualified therapists not only give counseling and guidance regarding effective communication techniques to parents and the child, but also to teachers to facilitate the child's learning at home and school.

Alternative Treatments for Bell's Palsy

There are several alternative treatments that Bell's palsy suffers can take to help alleviate their problem.

Methyl-Sulphonyl-Methane (MSM)

Methyl-Sulphonyl-Methane (MSM) is a sulphur-containing nutrient that can be found in a lot of the foods we eat. MSM acts as an anti-inflammatory and as such will be a benefit to Bells' palsy sufferers. By taking 500 mg of MSM three times a day will allow MSM to provide its anti-inflammatory properties for Bell's palsy sufferers.

Histamine

Although, if taken in large amounts histamine can be toxic to the body however if it is used in small amounts it is very effective in reducing inflammation and is beneficial for Bell's palsy sufferers. Histamine is not available in tablet form but the nutrient carnosine regulates the production of histamine and it is recommended that a daily dose of 100 mg will help Bell's palsy sufferers.

Adenosine Triphosphate (ATP)

The chemical Adenosine Triphosphate (ATP) has been proven to produce energy within cells. Experiments in combining ATP with the likes of vitamins B1, B2, B6 or B12 have shown that this combination can have an impact in the recovery from Bell's palsy. The results from the experiments showed that 100% of the patients who suffered with partial paralysis of the nerve, and approximately 87% of the patients who suffered with full paralysis recovered completely. Whereas approximately only 67% of the patients treated with steroids recovered.

Acetyl-L-Carnitine

The anti-inflammatory compound acetyl-L-Carnitine (ALC) has been found to improve the symptoms of Bell's palsy. ALC has been used for several neurological diseases such as nerve weakness, memory problems and nerve injuries. ALC has the ability to reduce any damage that is created by free radicals and it helps to preserve the production of energy within the nerve cells and as such stabilizes the nerve's membrane.

Chapter Seven: Correction with Surgery

Damage to the facial nerve affects how your face looks and also causes facial expressions (smiling, frowning, etc.) to become asymmetrical. There are various surgical options for the management of Bell's palsy. These include treatments for restoring the smile and facial balance, corrective surgeries such as face lifts, brow lifts and other muscle relaxing procedures.

These treatments are known to enhance the appearance of the face, but do not necessarily improve muscle function. It should be kept in mind that these procedures may not completely restore natural facial expressions or natural movement. But they can improve the patient's quality of life since the condition isn't as apparent.

Corrective surgery truly helps patients regain their confidence. Nevertheless, there are many people who have developed Bell's palsy and continue to live contentedly without any surgery. You also have to keep in mind that there are always risks associated with surgery. Let's take a look at some of these risks.

Oculoplastic Surgery

The foremost aim of this treatment is to enhance eye comfort and protect vision. Due to Bell's palsy, patients may experience eyelid retraction that can cause droopy eyebrows. This condition can be very painful as well. Oculoplastic surgery not only enhances the appearance of the eyes but is helpful in addressing problems such as watering of the eyes and incomplete eyelid closure.

This surgery involves a wide range of surgical procedures that involve the eyelids, orbit, face, and tear ducts. Therefore, this is the ideal type of surgery that people with Bell's palsy choose to undergo.

Eyelid Surgery

Most people with Bell's palsy have difficulty closing their eyelid. As previously discussed, this puts the eye at immense danger of infection or injury. Some patients may observe the improvement of eyelid function without any treatment. But those who experience lasting effects of Bell's palsy should not lose hope. Eyelid surgery helps these patients pull through the problem and protect their eye.

During Bell's palsy, the eyebrow may droop, and the upper eyelid may not close completely. Similarly, the lower eyelid may sag. This exposes your eye to the environment making it more susceptible to damage, discomfort and visual impairment. The main aim of eye surgery is to reduce discomfort. The surgery is also very effective in preserving vision.

As with any surgical procedure, there are certain risks associated with eye surgery. Remember, there are various other treatments, surgeries and therapies that are helpful for people suffering from Bell's palsy. You can discuss possible options with your doctor before making a final decision.

I've come across many people who live a very happy life even though they decided against having any surgical corrections. It really depends on what makes you happy as a person. If you can live with the fact that you have a droopy eye, then more power to you. However, if you don't want to deal with a droopy eye for life, you may choose to go under the knife.

Upper Eyelid Surgery

This surgery helps the upper lid cover more of the cornea and patients can close over 75% of their eye. Usually, it involves the surgical implantation of gold eyelid weights. The weights help the eyelid close with the help of gravity.

Gold eyelid weights can be implanted in an outpatient procedure. You can go back home the very same day. Once gold weights are attached to the eyelid, you can close the eyelid immediately. Minor bruising and swelling of the area is quite common, but it goes away in a few weeks.

There can be a slight bump on the eyelid where the weights are implanted. A qualified surgeon may place the gold implants in a place where they remain hidden. The reason gold weights are used is that the metal does not irritate a patient's skin. Gold weights are also safe to be used during an MRI.

The risk of upper eyelid surgery is that it can be difficult to control the position of the upper lid. If the eyelid still remains high, a repeat surgery may be required. Sometimes the weight may be too heavy, which will be seen as a bulky mass through the upper eyelid. The use of heavy weights can also blur your vision.

Lower Eyelid Surgery

Surgical correction of the lower eyelid is done to reduce watering and allow the eye to close more. The inner part of the lower eyelid on the affected side is stitched to the inner part of the upper eyelid. The procedure is short and can be performed under local anesthesia. However, the lower eyelid may droop or sag again in the future after surgery.

Lifting the central part of the lower eyelid requires a more complicated procedure. Also known as a scaffold procedure, it involves inserting tissue (from the ear or nose) into the center of the eyelid.

Eyebrow Surgery

An eyebrow lift is done in the area where the eyebrow is drooping. An incision is made above the eyebrow where tissue is removed, and the eyebrow is "fastened" to the deeper tissue of the forehead. Other eyebrow lifting methods involve the positioning of deep stitches that lift the eyebrow. The latter requires smaller incisions.

While eyebrow lifting surgeries are successful, the eyebrow may droop or fall again due to the continuing effect of gravity.

Eye Care during Bell's Palsy

Eye care is enormously essential in the early stages of Bell's palsy. Due to the damage to the facial nerve, certain functions such as blinking and eyelid movement are disturbed. Therefore, extra care must be taken to keep the eyes moist and protected from external debris and dust.

Symptoms and Effects on the Eye

The ability to blink, in many people, is adversely affected because of Bell's palsy. Patients are unable to close their eyes properly. The upper eyelid retraction and drooping of the lower lid causes incomplete closure of the eye. This results in excessive dryness.

Remember, if the eye is not lubricated, it could have severe implications such as exposure keratitis, permanent vision impairment and in some, cases blindness as well.

Usually, a normal person blinks every 5-7 seconds. Each time we blink, a film of tears spreads smoothly across the eye. However, Bell's palsy disrupts this function, and it becomes difficult for the eyelid on the affected side to shut completely. This exposes your eye to dryness and irritation. Remember, dry eyes are more susceptible to scratches from foreign objects. Deeper scratches can also cause scarring. Unfortunately, lasting damage to the cornea can also take place if the eye is not properly cared for.

Check Your Signs

If your eyes feel uncomfortable, do not overlook the issue. You may experience a stinging or burning sensation in the eye due to dryness.

Some individuals with Bell's palsy also experience crocodile tear syndrome. In this complication, the person tears excessively while eating. This is usually seen when a person is recovering but can also appear with the onset of the condition.

If your eyes feel dry, you may use artificial tears, commonly available at any drug store or supermarket. These eye drops will alleviate the stinging, burning sensation and also help maintain moisture in the eyes. It is advisable to look for preservative free eye drops. They have fewer additives and are usually labeled as non-allergic. You may use them 4-5 times a day at least, and of course each time your eyes feel dry.

During the night, it's important to keep the eye protected. Using an eye ointment along with a patch on the affected eye will help the eye remain moist while sleeping. You may even tape your eye shut so that it remains protected overnight.

If you have Bell's palsy, it is advised first to consult your doctor before starting with an eye care regime. You doctor may refer you to an optometrist if the eye symptoms get worse.

Cosmetic Reconstructive Options to Regain Facial Muscle Function

There are cosmetic reconstructive options that may help regain muscle function after Bell's palsy.

Brow-lifts, removal of excess eyelid skin, muscle relaxation procedures and facelifts are popularly used to improve facial appearance. Let's take a look at some of the more common procedures people opt for if they have Bell's palsy.

Facial Nerve Decompression

Decompression of the facial nerve relieves pressure and is usually done via a delicate microsurgical procedure. Pieces of the bone behind the ear are removed so that the nerve has adequate space to expand.

While this minor surgery is shown to produce a difference in some types of nerve damage, its use in Bell's palsy is still debatable.

Medical experts, in fact, regard facial nerve decompression in Bell's palsy as a highly controversial treatment. This is because there are serious medical risks involved. The most common complications include permanent damage to the 7th cranial nerve and hearing loss. In addition, there is no significant evidence that rates facial nerve compression a better alternative to standard medication.

If facial nerve decompression is to be done for Bell's palsy, it should be done within three weeks of the symptoms first appearing.

Statistics shows that once three weeks are over; there's no point in enduring the pain of surgery and the potential risks.

Hypoglossal and Facial Nerve Graft Repair

Nerve graft repairs can be used to improve muscle function as well as enhance facial appearance. However, these are complex surgical procedures and should only be considered after careful analysis of a patient's condition.

Grafting nerves seems like a good way to restore muscle appearance and function, but if not performed correctly, nerve graft repairs can leave a person with worse nerve paralysis than prior to surgery.

One type of nerve graft repair commonly employed involves connecting the hypoglossal nerve, i.e. the nerve that controls the tongue to the facial nerve. Once the surgery is done, the patient is taught how to move the face by carefully controlled tongue movements. Most people learn the technique gradually. This type of nerve graft is likely to end with a loss of sensation in the tongue.

Weakness in the tongue might also affect eating and swallowing.

Anesthesia Complications

Bell's palsy surgery itself is not usually very complex; however, some people may react adversely to anesthesia. They may face increased heart rate or high blood pressure when given anesthesia.

Bleeding Problems

Another possible complication of surgery is excessive bleeding. Certain patients may bleed more than others due to existing health conditions, which is why it is essential for the patient to consult their physician before they opt for corrective surgery. In the case of excessive bleeding, the patient may need a blood transfusion, which is prohibited in certain religions. So it is always wise to talk to your doctor beforehand to fully understand the risks of surgery.

Delayed Healing During Recovery

As human beings, we are all unique in the way we respond to surgery. The same goes with the recovery process. While some people have a swift recovery after surgery, others may take longer. If the recovery period is far beyond the normal range, it is bound to cause the patient some stress and anxiety.

Chapter Eight: Bell Palsy Exercises

It is best not to start any exercises until there are clear signs that the facial nerve is recovering and sending impulses to the muscles. Be sure to get approval from your doctor before starting an exercise regime.

Early Stages of Recovery

During the early stages on the road to recovery, facial massage is highly recommended.

Stage One

Gently massage the corner of the mouth, making your way up towards the ear with the help of your fingers. Then in a circular pattern, move the fingers down towards the jaw bone area. These circular movements are also beneficial for the forehead and chin area. Softly tap your skin with the help of your fingertips.

You may use a makeup brush or an electric toothbrush or simply your fingers for the following massage:

Massage your forehead upwards (in your hairline's direction) 3-4 times. Perform the same movements on your cheeks.

Stage Two

If you feel sore or experience spasms or stiffness at any particular point while carrying out your exercise regime, do not worry. It is advised to exert and hold pressure at that point for at least 15 seconds. This helps to relax the muscles.

Once the facial nerve has begun to recover, this set of exercises can be performed. It is always a good idea to perform these movements in front of a mirror. This way, you will be able to focus on the particular muscles. But bear in mind – never overexert your muscles. You may repeat these exercises 3-4 times a day for better results, however don't overdo it. As you can guess, good compliance is necessary to get a more fruitful outcome.

For the Eyebrows

Try raising your eyebrows slowly. Make sure that the corner of the mouth does not move upwards. Hold your pose for about 10 seconds, i.e. give a slight pause. Keep the muscles around the mouth extremely relaxed. Then repeat the movement.

If you have trouble moving the eyebrow on the affected side of the face, you may use your fingertips for assistance in the movement. Keeping your fingertips just above the eyebrows will help you raise them without trouble. This action can be repeated five times.

Once you have become accustomed to this, you may stop using your fingertips to raise your brows. Instead, start involving the forehead muscles in this activity.

Using the same guidelines as above, you may also wrinkle your forehead. It is a great way to relearn symmetrical facial movements. Now bring the eyebrows downwards and frown.

In the next exercise, do not move your eyebrow; instead open your eyes wide. This will help you assess if any improper muscle movements are taking place. If you feel you're not doing something right, seek help from a certified Bell's palsy therapist.

Other Exercises

For Your Eyes

Close your eyes slowly and make sure your eyebrow does not move downward. Place your fingers below and above your eye socket and stretch your eye slowly to a completely open position. Hold for a slow count of four. You may have to stretch a bit further and then pull your fingers back to close the eye.

The functionality of your eye is affected the most due to Bell's palsy. So while keeping the rest of the face as calm as possible, close one eye. You may also wink lightly with one eye and do it again with the other. Bear in mind, you should perform this movement very gently and as best as you can. Do not exert extra pressure on your eyes.

If you're not able to get it perfect the first time, there's no reason to worry. You can always seek help from a reputed Bell's palsy therapist to master the movement. If there's any significant pain or discomfort, consult your doctor immediately.

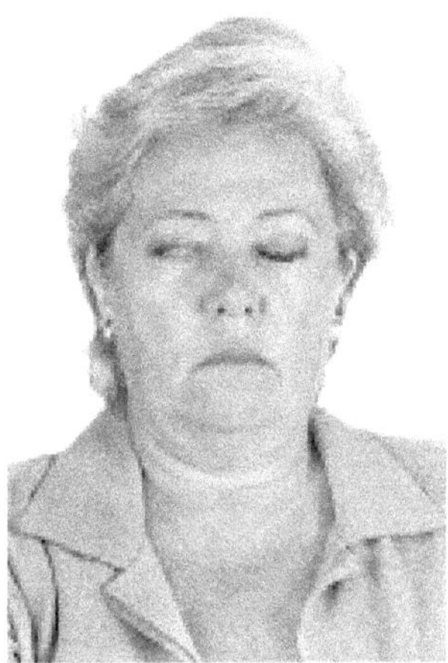

For the Nose

Wrinkle your nose and flare your nostrils as you may do when you smell something unpleasant. This will help use muscles around the nasal area.

Exercise for Cheeks

Puffing your cheeks is also a useful way to exercise the facial muscles. Using your fingers, seal your lips, and puff your cheeks out. Do this as symmetrically as you can. For best results, practice in front of a mirror. Blow your cheeks out at least five times.

With your fingers on your front teeth, gently move them along to the back of your teeth, to around where the molars are located. Molars are the largest teeth in your mouth. While doing so, stretch your cheeks and move your fingers underneath the gums. This is a good way to revive flexibility of the cheeks.

Restore Your Smile

A smile with your mouth closed is also an integral part of this exercise regime. Move the corners of your mouth to an outward position into a smile. To assist this movement, you may place your finger on the side of the mouth. And if it is difficult smiling on the affected side, you may place your hand over it and then push out and up into a smile.

It's a good idea to begin smiling, first without showing your teeth. After that, smile with your teeth showing.

Lip Movements

You may also move the corner of the mouth with your fingers and smoothly push outwards and say 'eee'. Similarly, position your fingers on each side of the mouth and push your lips outwards. And say 'ooo'. Now practice by saying these words repeatedly in this order: aaa...ooo…eee.

Practice pressing your lips together. Then pushing forward, pucker your lips as if though you're ready to give a kiss. Now release them. It is always a good idea to perform this exercise in front of a mirror.

Due to Bell's palsy, it becomes difficult to articulate some sounds. Practice speaking your vowels aloud to ease slurred speech. Focus on the lip movement of each vowel; a, e, i, o and u. Make sure you speak slowly and softly.

Chin Exercise

Jut your chin out the best you can. After that, using a firm circular motion, massage the nose, cheeks and chin. Continue the movement from the jaw line up to your ear. Use firm strokes but take care not to exert excess pressure.

Exercises to Assist Speech Therapy

Mouth isolation exercises can be very beneficial for patients suffering from Bell's palsy. These exercises can enhance their speech quality and hence, make them feel more confident. These basic movements aim to improve the tone of the affected facial muscles, which helps the patient speak more clearly.

Warm-up Activities

1. This regime begins with simple warm up activities such as flaring and constricting the nostrils. You are then required to curl the upper lip up. After that, you will practice to raise and protrude the upper lip. Another easy way to practice lip movements is to pucker the lips (like you're kissing someone) and then attempt to whistle.

2. Other exercises can also help improve facial function and will assist you in speaking clearly. For example, you can try smiling without showing teeth first and then smile with teeth. To help with the exercise, try to perform these actions in front of a mirror. You should also attempt to repeat words that have the letters B and P.

3. Rehearsing resistance exercises is also necessary to assist the toning of facial muscles that eventually makes speaking easier. For that, place your thumb and the index finger near the corner of the lips. Now try smiling as wide as you can. The thumb and index finger will offer resistance. Repeat this exercise at least ten times.

4. Bell's palsy can cause your cheek to droop, which makes it difficult to talk. Talking over the phone can be particularly troublesome because of it. You can rest your hand against your cheek when opening your mouth to speak. This may help you sound better and provide support to the 'floppy' cheek.

5. You should also try to stimulate the droopy cheek through a tender massage. It can be performed just by massaging your

cheeks in a circular motion with the help of your fingertips. All you have to do is make large strokes starting from the mouth towards the ear. You may also use ice cubes by holding them against your face, from the lips across your cheek to the ears.

Specialized Facial Exercise Program to Improve Speech

The following is another simple, specialized facial exercise program that can help improve your speech. These exercises involve strengthening the muscles in your tongue, lips and jaw.

Exercises for the Tongue

Stage One

Stick your tongue out as far as possible and hold this position for about 5 seconds. Next, do the exact opposite, i.e. retract your tongue back inside and hold it close to the 'roof' of your mouth. Relax for 3 to 5 seconds and then move your tongue up and down, side to side with your mouth closed. You can also try pushing your tongue against your teeth followed by rest.

Stage Two

In the second stage, we will be adding more resistance to the exercises.

Stick your tongue out and press it down gently using the back of a spoon while you try to lift it. Next, repeat the same exercise, but try to move your tongue to the left and then the right.

In the final exercise, place your index finger on your affected cheek about one inch from the corner of your mouth. Now try to push this finger using your tongue from the inside of your mouth.

You can do five to eight repetitions of each tongue exercise.

Exercises for the Jaws

In this exercise, you have to stretch your jaw the same way you stretched your tongue. First, open your mouth as wide as you can. Now move your lower jaw first to the left and then to the right. In the next step, try moving your jaw in a circular motion. Try doing five repetitions of each movement. You may provide resistance with your hand to help tone your jaw muscles.

Exercising Your Lips

As you know, the movement of your lips plays an important part in the way you speak. Start the exercise by smiling with your mouth closed for about five seconds. Next, hold your lips in a kissing pose for another five seconds.

Now, try combining the movements, i.e. smile and then pucker your lips. Make sure you fully use your facial muscles.

Next, squeeze your lips using a tongue depressor (the flat wooden stick with rounded corners the doctor inserts in your mouth to check your throat) or any other similar tool. Then try to pull your lips out. Finally, repeat each lip exercise five times.

Helpful Illustrations

Here are some illustrations that you will find useful.

Eye Exercises

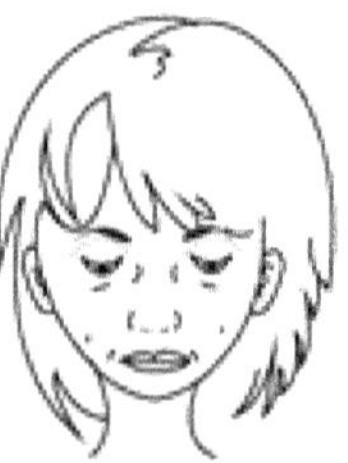

Look down

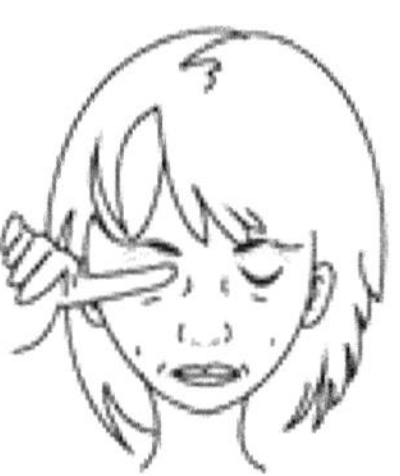

Lightly place the back of your index finger on your eyelid to keep your eye closed

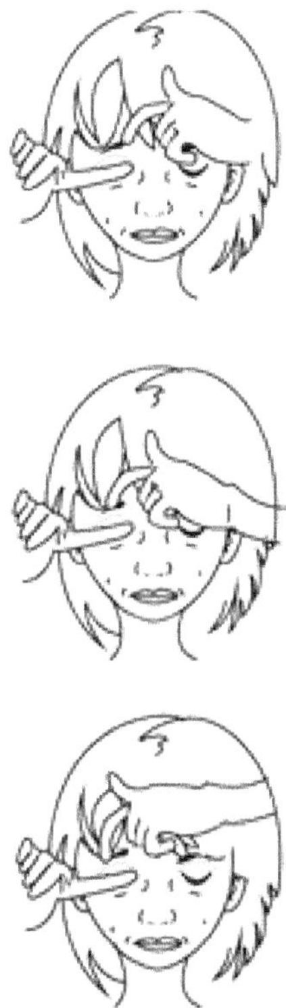

Using your opposite hand gently stretch your eyebrow up, working your finger across the brow line. This helps relax your eyelid and prevents it from becoming stiff

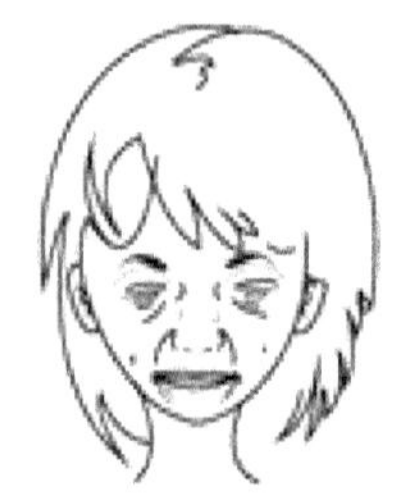

Now close your eyes tightly

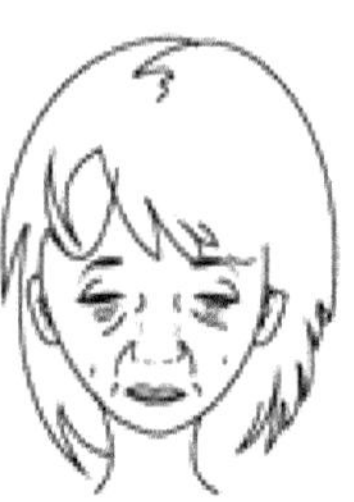

Open your eyes and squint as if you were looking at the sun

Face Exercises

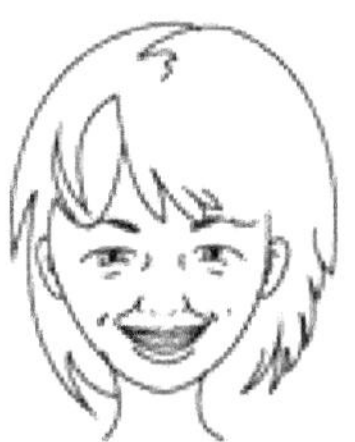

Turn the corners of the mouth up

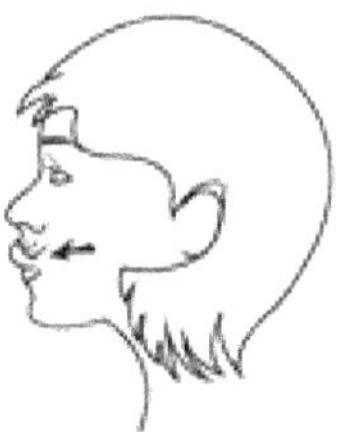

Push the upper lip forward

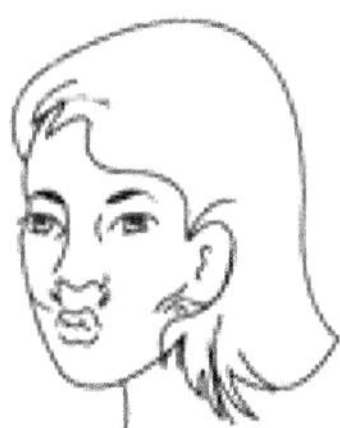

Suck in the cheeks and push the lips forward

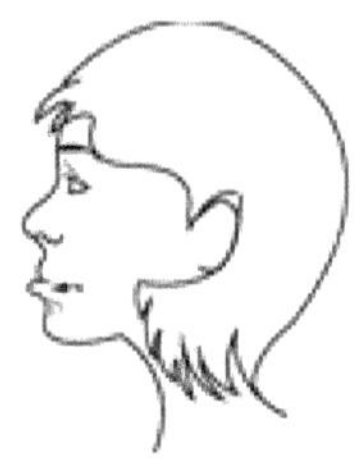

Push the lower lip forward

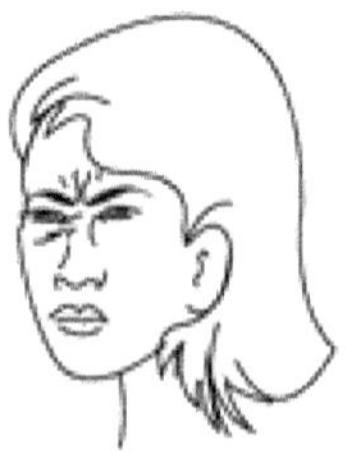

Bring the eyebrows together
in a frown

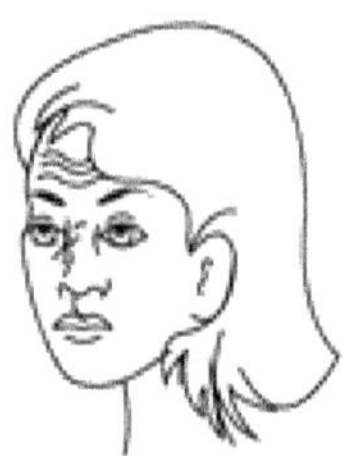

Raise the eyebrows

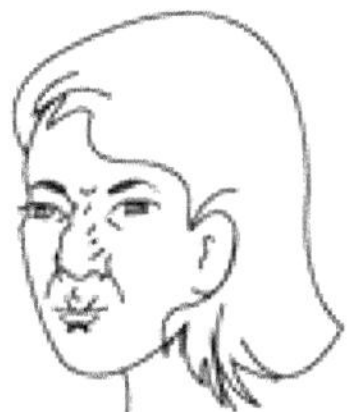

wrinkle the nose

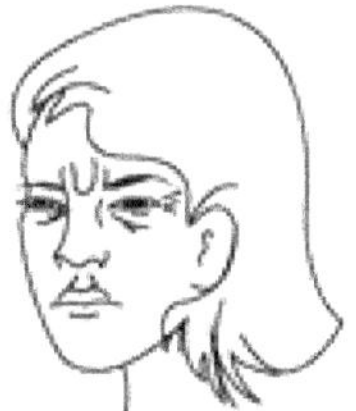

Squint the eyes tightly

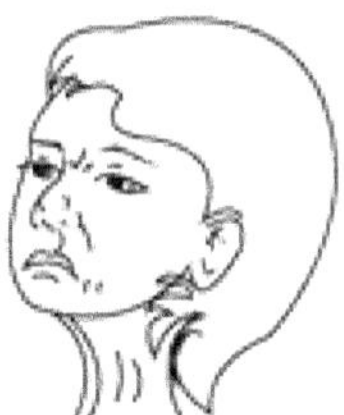

Turn the corners of the mouth down
and tighten the muscles on the front of the neck

Chapter Nine: Useful Diet and Lifestyle Considerations

Apart from psychological issues such as depression and mood swings, Bell's palsy can cause various physiological issues that impair many patients' lives.

Eating and drinking are some of the daily tasks that become complicated to perform. Another great concern is the lack of oral hygiene. Most patients find it difficult to brush their teeth properly, especially on the side of the face that is affected by the condition. They experience difficulty opening their mouth and suffer from nagging problems such as food spilling from their mouth and dry mouth.

Apart from the difficulty in maintaining oral hygiene, patients also complain of changes in the quantity of saliva that is produced.

Patients, who experience decreased production of saliva, are susceptible to tooth decay and gum disease. Remember, saliva has a crucial responsibility of protecting your teeth.

Taking Care of Your Oral Health

Dentists emphasize the significance of flossing apart from brushing your teeth twice a day. For good oral hygiene, a good quality mouthwash should also be included in your list of essentials. After every meal, it is advised to rinse the mouth thoroughly with the mouthwash as directed so that any food residue and bacteria is removed. Also don't forget to floss so that any unwanted particles in between your teeth are removed. This will prevent bad breath.

What If I Use Dentures?

Due to Bell's palsy, the ability to chew food is also compromised. This is mainly because of the loss of muscle tone on the paralyzed side of the face. Unfortunately, the condition can cause problems for those who wear dentures. Simply put, Bell's palsy can lead to unstable dentures. If you have false teeth, you may have to pay extra attention to dental hygiene and must clean the dentures every day.

If you are undergoing any procedure, it is advisable to postpone the dental treatment until you have recovered from the condition. The reason is to avoid any fatigue and stress. However, if the treatment cannot be rescheduled or delayed, make sure you inform your dentist about your condition and the medication that you are taking.

Dentists usually use special equipment such as a rubber bite or tongue retractor for patients who have Bell's palsy. These tools are used to control the parts of the tongue and mouth affected by the condition. Patients may find it difficult to keep the mouth open for very long. Also, they may have issues swallowing and controlling their tongue, which is why this equipment is used.

Here are some tips to prevent dental issues if you wear dentures:

1. The use of a mouthwash should be a vital part of your daily routine.
2. In order to avoid any sores, it is always a good idea to rinse your mouth with warm water once you have finished your meal.
3. Always take small bites of food and try to involve both sides of the mouth while chewing.
4. If you are experiencing major difficulty while swallowing food, you should have semi solid food such as pudding, yogurt, or jelly. Also, foods that have texture such as oatmeal are easier to eat.
5. You may also use straws to assist you when drinking. However, you may have to practice drinking through the straw correctly. Make sure you keep the straw in the center of the mouth while drinking. You may also support your lips with your fingertips so that your mouth forms a seal.

Taking Care of a Dry Mouth

Damage to the facial nerve as a result of Bell's palsy causes changes in several normal physiological functions. One such problem is the production of saliva.

Salivary glands are stimulated by the 7th cranial nerve. But when the nerve becomes inflamed or irritated, it adversely affects the functioning of the salivary glands. Swelling and irritation of the nerve causes decreased saliva production. This results in an extreme dry mouth for some patients. The condition is also called xerostomia. This leads to other issues such as problems eating properly or throat disorders.

Quite often, we do not understand the importance of saliva. However, it is worth mentioning that saliva plays a crucial role in keeping your mouth healthy. It performs various functions such as preventing sores and mouth ulcers due to its lubricating properties. It also helps us with our ability to taste food. It contains essential enzymes that are integral for the digestive process. Remember, it is only because of saliva that we can chew food thoroughly since it helps break down food.

Saliva production also helps prevent tooth loss and tooth decay, keeping the mouth clean and protected from plaque. With decreased saliva to wash away bacteria, patients with dry mouth are vulnerable to oral infections and tooth decay.

Treating Dry Mouth

There are various ways through which you can treat dry mouth caused by Bell's palsy.

a. As discussed in the previous section, good oral hygiene is really important if you have Bell's palsy. So brush regularly twice a day and use dental floss. It is recommended that you see your dentist every four months.

b. You should take frequent sips of water or other sugar-free drinks. One great idea is to have a bottle of water with you most of the time like athletes and fitness buffs. You can also keep a water bottle beside your bed when you go to sleep. But avoid having drinks that are very sugary. Drinks loaded with sugar may further aggravate or worsen dental complications.

c. If you experience an extremely dry mouth, you should strictly avoid alcohol and caffeine. Both alcohol and caffeine have dehydrating characteristics due to their diuretic properties. And dehydration could cause severe problems if you are already suffering from a dry mouth. So it's better to increase the intake of water rather than consume these drinks. You may have decaffeinated tea if you desire.

d. If you have problems chewing food because of a dry mouth and other Bell's palsy symptoms, you can increase the quantity of sauce, broth and gravy in your meals. This will help moisten the food make it easier for you to chew and swallow. It is recommended that you avoid dry foods and bread.

e. Apart from sugary foods, it is also advised to restrict acidic foods such as citric fruits. Apart from this, you should avoid other substances such as cigarettes that are known to increase dryness of the mouth.

f. There are certain products in the market that act as oral moisturizing agents. They include topical gels, toothpaste and mouthwash specifically designed to reduce dry mouth. You may ask your doctor to recommend a suitable product. Use the products strictly as directed.

Nutritional Requirements for Children

Since children suffering from Bell's palsy often have a compromised immune system, it is important that you pay attention to what they eat.

Good nutrition, as suggested by the American Dietetic Association, can rebuild and strengthen a child's immune system.

Kids often prefer to eat semi-solid foods such as pudding, jelly and yogurt and you may add a multivitamin liquid preparation to them after consulting a certified pediatrician. It is better to stick to semi-solid and liquid foods if the child is having problems swallowing.

Make sure you include the following food groups in the kid's diet plan.

1. Fruits: Try to include at least two servings of fruit per day. One serving here refers to one piece of fruit or ½ cup canned fruit or ¾ cup fruit juice or ¼ cup dried fruit. It's always best to include fresh produce in your child's diet plan.

2. Milk and Dairy: Kids might not be fond of dairy products but be sure to include two servings of dairy per day. One serving includes 2 oz. cheese or 1 cup of milk/yogurt. Please check with a doctor if your child is lactose intolerant.

3. Protein: Cooked lean meat, poultry or fish, beans, eggs and peanut butter can be used as ideal protein sources. Kids require two servings (85g each) of the protein group.

4. Whole grains and vegetables are also valuable options that cannot be ignored. You can include six servings of the grain group and three servings of veggies throughout the day. ½ cup of chopped raw or cooked vegetables or one cup of raw, leafy vegetables is counted as one serving. One slice of bread or ½ cup cooked rice/pasta, or ½ cup ready-to-eat cereal is one serving of the grains group.

5. Fatty and sugary food should be limited as much as possible.

What Should I Eat?

There isn't any particular food or special cuisine that you need to follow. But as with any other medical complication, it is better if you stick to a balanced diet plan during facial paralysis. Bell's palsy without a doubt takes a toll on your immune system, so you need to fulfill your body's nutritional needs. Remember, even small dietary changes can be extremely useful in speeding up the nerve healing process.

a. Foods rich in vitamins, minerals and fiber should be an essential part of your diet while recovering from this condition. If you are suffering from Bell's palsy, be sure to eat plenty of fresh fruits, whole grains and leafy, green vegetables such as kale and spinach.

b. You can also choose low-fat dairy products and lean meat options such as chicken and turkey. Seafood, in fact, makes an excellent choice and definitely deserves a place in your diet plan. Fish are rich sources of vitamin B12 that is known to boost nerve growth and repair.

c. Seafood such as oysters and shellfish contain copper that is vital to nerve health. Copper can also be found in cocoa and beans. It's also a good idea to include cod liver oil in your diet; studies show that cod liver oil is very helpful in repairing the damaged myelin sheath.

d. Also, try your best to avoid processed foods and foods having high saturated fat or sugar content. While sugar and saturated fats might not cause your facial palsy symptoms to worsen, they do slow down the healing process. Medical research shows that foods high in saturated fats (bad fats) can disrupt the normal healing process and prevent your body from functioning at its optimal level.

e. One of the most essential nutrients that need to be part of your diet plan are vitamin B12 and vitamin B6, which we covered previously. They are extremely beneficial in encouraging nerve repair and growth. You may find a lot of supplements in the market, but nothing can substitute consumption of the nutrients through the diet directly.

f. You will find a wide range of vitamins and minerals in seafood such as shellfish, crabs, tuna and salmon as well as dark leafy greens such as spinach. Cauliflower, peppers and broccoli are also rich sources of vitamin B6 which is another important nutrient that you should not forget to consume.

g. Remember, your diet plan will be incomplete without the inclusion of Zinc. Firstly, it is known to strengthen the immune system which is necessary to speed up the Bell's palsy healing process. If you recall the causes of Bell's palsy, viruses that cause cold and flu are known to trigger the condition. Hence, it is vital to consume nutrients that can help the body defend against nasty viruses.

h. Try to include a lot of beans, fortified cereals, chickpeas, oysters and chicken in your diet - they all are rich sources of zinc.

Foods to Avoid

Saturated Fats

If you want assist your facial palsy recovery, make sure you stay away from bad saturated fats. Remember, bad fats are threatening for your heart. These fats can be found in red meat and dairy products with high-fat content such as high-fat cheeses and butter. It is recommended that you focus more on low-fat dairy products such as skimmed milk. And while choosing animal meat, go for 'leaner' options such as chicken, turkey and low-fat cuts of beef and pork.

Refined Carbohydrates

Refined or processed sugars, unfortunately, are one of the strongest irritants of the nervous system. This means sodas, pastries, candies and everything that is high in refined carbohydrates, can have detrimental effects on your recovery. Try to eliminate as much white bread and pastas as you can from your diet as they are also known to worsen nerve health.

Foods to Include In Your Diet

Folic Acid

You should eat more of the foods that are rich in folic acid and vitamin B12. Both nutrients are essential for the maintenance of healthy nervous system function and adequate repair of nerve insulating material, i.e. myelin sheath. Folic acid in particular is significant in the regeneration of the 7th cranial nerve. Food sources you should also incorporate into your diet include nuts, seeds, eggs, animal liver, whole grains, and beans.

Anti-inflammatory Herbs

Adding herbs such as turmeric and ginger in your diet is a great way to reduce inflammation of the facial nerve. You can also add green tea to your diet plan as it is known to protect the myelin sheath.

Vitamin C

Vitamin C is one of the most potent natural immune system boosters, so get your hands on those juicy lemons and oranges. You can also try guava and grapefruits to ensure that your body gets an adequate supply of vitamin C. Surprisingly; generous intake of this vitamin also protects the myelin sheath as this nutrient is also a powerful anti-inflammatory and anti-oxidizing agent.

Vitamin A and D are valuable supports for your immune system. You can go for orange fruits and veggies such as papaya, carrots and oranges that are rich sources of vitamin A. Cod liver oil is another good source of vitamin A, D and essential fatty acids.

Essential Fatty Acids

Your brain is composed of 60% fat, and you require good fats like fat omega-3 and omega-6 to maintain a healthy brain. Be sure you include rich sources of omega-6 in your diet such as chicken, fish, walnuts and extra virgin olive oil. Both omega-3 and omega-6 fatty acids help reduce nerve inflammation and improve electrical transmission.

Fruits

Bananas are an excellent choice as they are packed with several nutrients like potassium. Citrus fruits, grapes and tropical fruits, not only are an ideal substitute for sweets and candies but are full of powerful immune boosters especially Vitamin C, which is essential for those suffering from Bell's palsy. Eating a cup of blueberries daily can also alleviate symptoms of facial palsy as the berries have incredible anti-inflammatory and healing properties.

Here's another friendly reminder: Try to eat raw veggies and fresh fruits as they are loaded with vital nutrients. You also need to drink plenty of water as it is one of the best conductors of electrical impulses. Also try substituting sugary drinks and caffeine with plain water and try to drink at least 2 liters of water per day.

Chapter Ten: Have Your Say

So this brings us to the completion of the book. We have discussed a wide variety of aspects related to Bell's palsy, starting from what it is, what the symptoms are, how it's caused, who is most likely to be affected by it, and finally, how you can treat it.

It has been a long, but hopefully, beneficial journey through which you have learned about the important aspects of Bell's palsy and how it affects lives. To many it may not seem like a serious condition, however, to those who have it or have had it, it can be quite debilitating.

You may experience low self-esteem, lose the confidence to mingle with others, and eventually end up isolating yourself. But again, this condition in the majority of instances is temporary and treatable. So don't let it take over your life.

With the help of this book on Bell's palsy, you can be on your way to living a happier and healthier life.

I truly hope that you enjoyed reading the book. My intention was to help every Bell's palsy patient so that they fully understand the condition and that they are fully aware of the treatment options available to them. If you have any feedback, comments or suggestions, please do not hesitate to get in touch. You may contact me at **bellspalsy@alanmcdonald.org**. It's been a pleasure writing this book, and I would love to hear from you.

If you enjoyed the book and found it useful, may I ask that you please leave me a 5-star review if you purchased the book via Amazon. I'd highly appreciate the gesture, and it would really help validate the many hard hours I have spent compiling this book.

Alan McDonald

Index

Index

Notes

Notes

www.ingramcontent.com/pod-product-compliance
Lightning Source LLC
LaVergne TN
LVHW010951100826
845153LV00002B/196

* 9 7 8 0 9 9 3 1 6 2 2 1 3 *